marathon
training

marathon training

Get to the Start Line Strong and Injury-free

nikalas cook

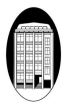

ROBERT HALE • LONDON

© Nikalas Cook 2012
First published in Great Britain 2012

ISBN 978-0-7090-9329-9

Robert Hale Limited
Clerkenwell House
Clerkenwell Green
London EC1R 0HT

www.halebooks.com

The right of Nikalas Cook to be identified as
author of this work has been asserted by him
in accordance with the Copyright, Designs and
Patents Act 1988

All images © the author, except where stated

A catalogue record for this book is available from the British Library

2 4 6 8 10 9 7 5 3 1

Typeset by Eurodesign
Printed in China

A huge thank you to my wife Lissa for her
support while writing this book and during all
of my madcap adventures, training and races.
Standing at the bottom of a hill with spare bike wheels
in the pouring rain is the definition of true love.

Contents

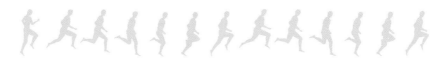

Introduction

Inspired by Pheidippides' fabled run from the Battle of Marathon to Athens in 490 BC, the marathon was one of the original modern Olympic events in 1896. The iconic 42.195 km (26 miles and 385 yards) was first run at the 1908 London Olympics. The rather arbitrary distance came about owing to the race having to finish under the Royal Box, so you can blame the Royal Family for the extra distance you have to run. It wasn't until 1921, though, that the distance became standardized, and for the first seven Olympic Games there were six different marathon distances between 40 and 42.74 km.

The real 'marathon boom' for the masses occurred in the 1980s and the major city centre marathons now attract runners in their thousands. Huge amounts of money are raised for charity, and every single participant will have an experience that will stay with them for a lifetime.

Every year, the day after a big city centre marathon, thousands of inspired people don an old T-shirt and a battered pair of plimsolls, do a few limbering-up exercises against their neighbour's fence and set out for their first training run. Unfortunately, for the majority of people this first foray into running ends a couple of hundred yards up the road in a wheezing red-faced heap, a stagger home and the conclusion that they're just not a runner. Some brave souls manage to plod along for 10 or 20 minutes but the muscle soreness the next day consigns many off them to the running scrap heap. A small minority develop a regular running habit but, en route to 26.2-mile glory, boredom, the British winter and the physiotherapist's couch all claim their victims. Recent studies show a 50–60 per cent injury rate in the year building up to a

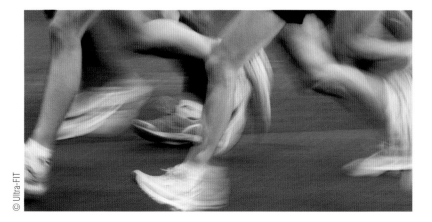

marathon, so something must be going wrong somewhere. The most obvious culprit has to be the running intensive, high volume and unfocused training plans that people are following.

Running is deeply rooted in our evolutionary past, and we're all hard-wired and anatomically adapted to be long-distance runners. Some of us are more gifted, with longer limbs or larger lungs, but with a planned and progressive approach to training, if you can run 10 yards, you can run a marathon. The classic mistake people make is assuming they can already run. If you're already active and play sports that involve running this may be true, but if you're sedentary and haven't really run since the hell of school cross-country, then should it really be a surprise that you can't just get up and go out for a run? Equally, running is a learnt skill with a number of key technical pointers. You wouldn't start training for a Channel swim without learning to swim properly, so why start training for a marathon before learning to run properly? Running with poor technique makes you more prone to injury, less efficient and slower. You only have to take a look at the horror show of running styles at any local park to realize that correct running technique shouldn't be taken for granted. As well as learning to run, preparing your body for running is essential. In our modern lives, the majority of our time is spent sitting down, meaning that important running muscles don't fire correctly, are chronically shortened or are wasted and weak. Other muscles try to take up the slack, but this just leads to imbalances and injuries. A balanced strengthening and stretching routine to address these issues is an essential part of a successful running plan.

Many marathon training plans make the error of prescribing far too much running. Although it may seem that more is better, in reality this is a guaranteed route to injury. Biomechanically gifted elite athletes can just about get away with these massive training volumes, but even they are constantly walking an injury knife edge. Five or six running sessions per week are unnecessary, and you're far more likely to arrive at the start line fit, strong and well by adopting a more varied and less running intensive plan. Three running sessions per week combined with cross-training sessions – including, for example, strength work, cycling and swimming – is a much more balanced, effective and body friendly approach. Another standard in most marathon training plans are the three- to four-hour, 18 to 22-mile training runs at weekends. Four to six of these are usually programmed into the final couple of months of most plans, so it's no wonder that this is when most people pick up injuries. These runs are also so taxing on the body that consistent training during the week is practically impossible. Yes, if you get through these runs unscathed, they'll give you confidence, but the risk of injury, impact on your training and demands on your time totally devalue them. The longest runs in this plan are two and a half hours. This length strikes a perfect balance between getting you prepared for the big day, not trashing you for the rest of the week and not leaving you injured. You'll obviously be running for longer on marathon day, but you'll have more than enough strength and stamina to cover the extra distance, and you won't be carrying an injury.

Training for a marathon is something that should never be rushed. Plans that fast-track people from non-runners to a full marathon in three months are unrealistic, irresponsible and dangerous. For every runner who makes it through, there will be 10 others lining the pockets of physios or vowing never to run again. The absolute minimum amount of time a non-runner should expect to take is 28 weeks, or seven months. While this might seem a long time, it's necessary to allow the physiological adaptations of your body's energy and musculoskeletal systems to take place. However, as you progress through the plan, there are significant goals and milestones along the way to keep you interested and motivated. If you're already a runner you can enter the programme at the point suited to your experience, but if you've been plagued by injury, or struggle to go beyond a certain point, it'd be worth going back a level.

KEY POINTS

✓ High volume, exclusively running-focused plans result in high injury rates.

✓ If you can run 10 yards, you can run a marathon.

✓ Running well is a skill that has to be learnt.

✓ We have to prepare and strengthen our bodies to run and undo the damage of sitting.

✓ Cross-training builds balanced fitness and an injury resistant body.

✓ Consistency of training is more important than massively long weekend runs.

✓ You can't rush marathon training.

HOW TO USE THIS BOOK

For a novice runner, the ideal way to use this book is to find a marathon a minimum of 28 weeks away and work through the whole plan towards it. I'd strongly suggest adding four to five 'buffer weeks' to allow for illness, busy work periods or any of those other life niggles that get in the way of running. If you're working towards specific events for the intermediary distances (5 km, 10 km and half marathon), allow at least the suggested number of weeks for that stage of the plan, but if you end up with extra time, repeat the penultimate week of the level to fill the additional weeks before moving on to the final week. If you are ill or miss a significant number of sessions in a week, don't just move on to the next week, but repeat the week you failed to complete.

For more experienced runners, who are able to run for 30 minutes or more, rather than leaping ahead to Level 3 or 4, you should go back to Level 2. This might feel as though you're taking a step backwards, especially if you've already run a 10 km event or a half or even full marathon, but establishing the functional strength foundation is an investment worth making. This is particularly important if you've suffered from injuries when training for races in the past.

CHAPTER 1

Level 1: Weeks 1–8

Preparing to run and your first 5 km

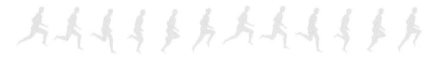

Strength Training

WHY IS IT NECESSARY?

If running is one of the most natural activities we can take part in and we evolved to do it, why do so many runners pick up injuries? If our bodies are adapted to running, why do we need to do any special preparation to run? One of the answers is that although we might be the same 'running animal' as our mammoth-hunting ancestors, our modern lifestyle isn't what we evolved for. This means that all the wonderful anatomical features that should allow us to run effortlessly for hours on end are underused, compromised, weakened and ineffective. When we do throw ourselves overenthusiastically into a running training programme, our bodies simply can't cope. A good analogy would be keeping a high performance racing car garaged for years and then, on the first turn of the key and without any servicing, expecting it to post a record lap on a racetrack.

One of the biggest contributing factors to our bodies' diminished ability to run is the amount of time we spend sitting. Think about it. Working at your desk, driving your car or sitting watching the TV, 12 hours on your backside each day isn't beyond the realms of possibility. We didn't evolve as sitters, we evolved as upright movers, hunting, gathering and avoiding being eaten. Sitting causes all sorts of problems. Key muscle groups for running such as our hamstrings and hip flexors tighten and weaken. Supportive muscles in the core and buttocks that are vital for strong, injury free running switch off and waste away. When we then go out and run, other muscles and tissues take up the strain to compensate for the weakened ones that are supposed to be doing the job, but this just compounds the problem and sets you up for injury woes.

The strengthening routine that'll be an integral part of your preparation and training is designed to undo the damage that sitting has done, switch on and strengthen your running muscles and make sure you start running correctly and strongly. Many of the exercises in the strengthening routine are ones that you'd typically find in the rehab routines that phyios prescribe for injured runners. As far as I'm concerned, that's closing the stable door after the horse has bolted, and it's obviously far better to get strong for running and not get injured at all.

As well as leg strengthening exercises that have an obvious relationship to running, the core-strengthening movements included are vital for providing a strong running platform and safeguarding you against non-running injuries and mishaps. This 'Robust or Bust' philosophy to conditioning was coined by a good friend of mine and top sports physio, Tim Deykin. He was working with the British slalom canoeing squad and noticed that, although they were super strong in their boats, they were relatively weak outside them and prone to injuries in everyday life. This is another reason why strengthening work has to be more than an optional extra in a marathon programme. You're investing a staggering amount of time and effort in your training and definitely don't want a silly niggle picked up gardening or doing DIY to ruin it all. Building a great all-round strength base is the best insurance policy you can take out against this.

The strengthening routine is easy to do at home or in the gym with the minimum amount of kit. All you'll need is:

✓ An exercise mat.
✓ A Swiss/stability ball.
✓ Adjustable dumbbells or a selection of dumbbell weights.

Exercise	Reps	Sets	Recovery
Single-legged squat	10 (each leg)	3	Recover while other leg is working
Single-legged deadlift	10 (each leg)	3	Recover while other leg is working
Walking lunge with twist	10 (each leg)	3	60 seconds
Calf raises	20 (each leg)	3	Recover while other leg is working
Ball hamstring curl	15	3	60 seconds
One-legged dynamic bridge	15–20 (each leg)	2	Recover while other leg is working
Roll-outs	10–15	2	60 seconds
Oblique plank	30–60 seconds each side	2	Recover while other side is working

EXERCISE DESCRIPTIONS

Single-legged squat: An excellent movement for developing running-specific strength, and for targeting those vital glutes:

Single-legged squat finish

- ✓ Go as deep as you can manage and tap your hind foot on the floor.
- ✓ Bend forwards and reach out with your arms to assist balance.
- ✓ Focus on engaging your butt muscles.
- ✓ As you progress, deepen the movement by standing on a step or bench.

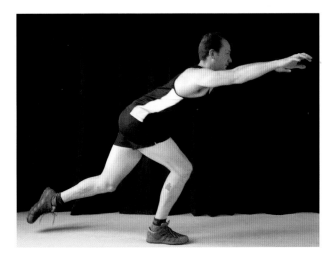

Single-legged
deadlift start

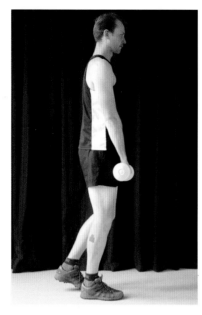

Single-legged deadlift: Another single-legged movement, but this time working predominately on the hamstrings and lower back:

- ✓ Keep a slight bend in the standing leg.
- ✓ Keep your head up and your spine neutral.
- ✓ Lower the dumbbell to just in front of the standing foot.

Single-legged
deadlift finish

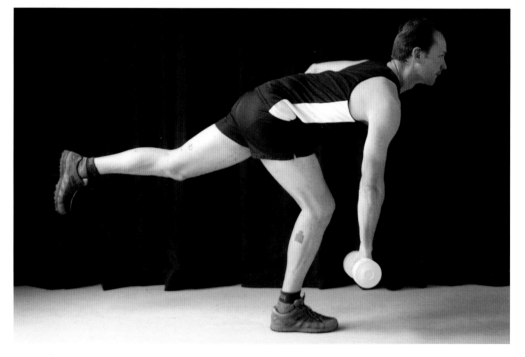

Walking lunge with twist: More single-legged movement, and the twist helps to develop lateral strength and stability:

✓ Step slightly outside your centre line to give a more stable platform for the twist.
✓ Make sure the twist is slow and controlled.
✓ Hold a dumbbell or medicine ball to increase the intensity.

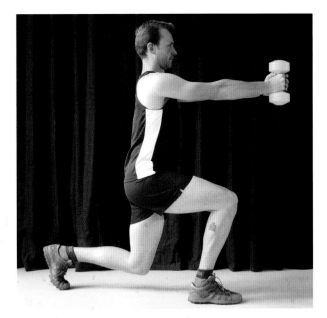

Walking lunge with twist start

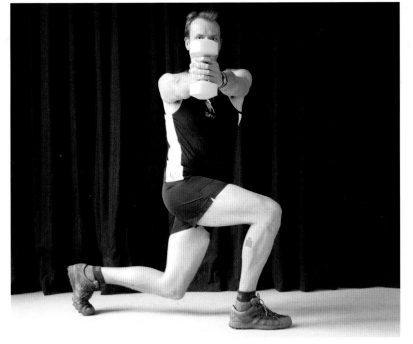

Walking lunge with twist finish

Calf raises: Your calves and Achilles' tendon are particularly vulnerable to injury, so some strengthening is strongly advised:

✓ Try to do one leg at a time to identify any discrepancies.
✓ Standing on a step or bench is more beneficial than using a seated station.
✓ Work through a full range of motion, from a deep stretch with the heel fully down to full extension right up on tiptoe.

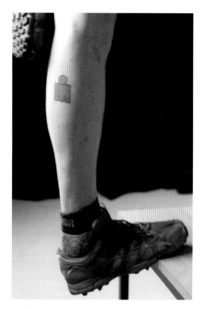

Calf raise start

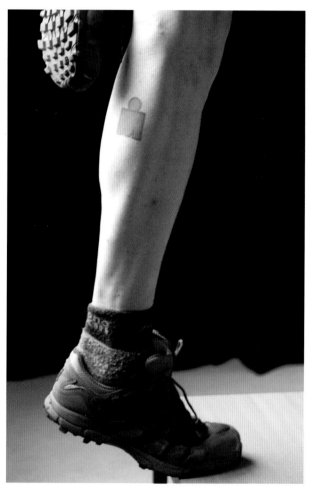

Calf raise finish

Ball hamstring curl: As well as hitting the hamstrings, an excellent movement for building core stability and strength:

✓ Keep your hips high and butt muscles clenched.
✓ Work in a slow, controlled and balanced manner.
✓ Aim to progress to performing the movement single-legged.

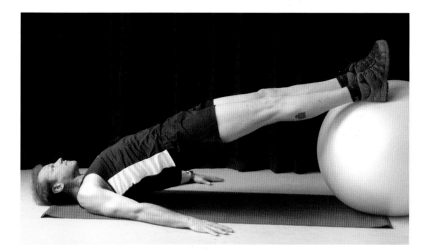

Ball hamstring curl
start

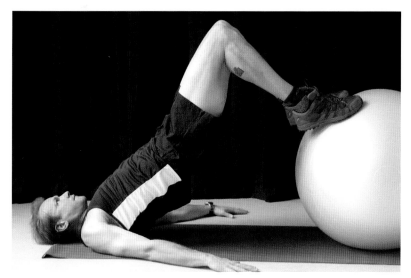

Ball hamstring curl
finish

One-legged dynamic bridge: Following on from the work on the ball, this again will hit your backside and hamstrings:

✓ As you lift your hips, squeeze your bum.
✓ Keep the non-supporting leg extended, pointing with the toes and the thigh parallel to the supporting leg.
✓ Lower to the point where your bum just touches the floor, and then drive straight back up.

One legged dynamic bridge finish

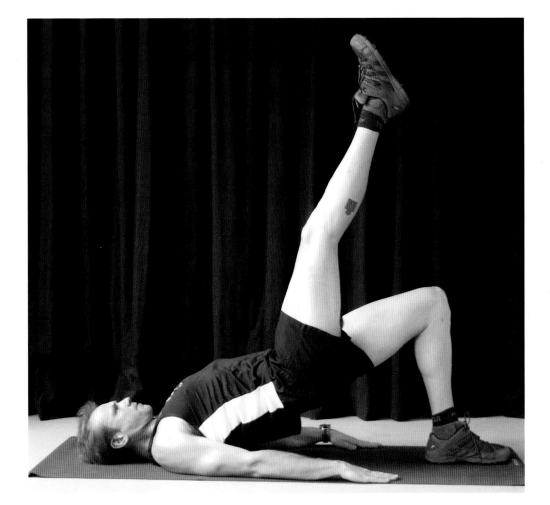

Roll-outs: The deep stabilizer muscles of your trunk are essential for avoiding excessive body roll when running. This movement targets them in a dynamic way:

✓ Maintain a neutral spine throughout with no hint of hyperextension.
✓ Don't roll too far; keep in control of the movement.
✓ Strongly contract your abdominal muscles throughout.

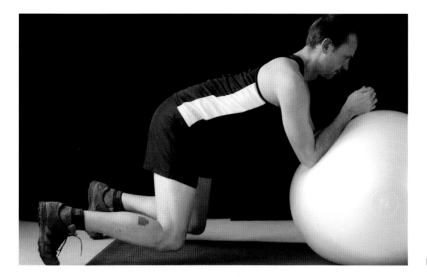

Roll out start

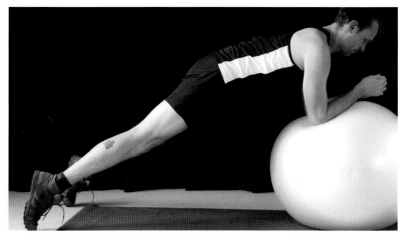

Roll out finish

Oblique plank: A second movement aimed at delivering a stable and strong trunk:

✓ Keep your head up, and avoid sagging or lifting the hips.
✓ Reach high with the extended hand, and open your chest to almost the point of overbalancing backwards.
✓ Stop the 'rep' when your form deteriorates.

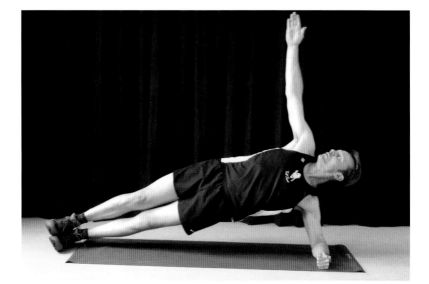

Oblique plank

Stretching and Running

Stretching and its relationship to running is a controversial subject. Runners tend to fall into one of three camps. The first are the stretching evangelists who'll take every opportunity to contort themselves into extreme stretches and will wax lyrical about the benefits of stretching. At the other end of the spectrum are the complete non-stretchers who'll scoff at that 'stretching nonsense' and whose idea of post-running recovery is a cup of tea. In the middle tend to be the majority of runners. They'll have a vague notion about some stretches, usually do a few after a run, and sometimes include a few as they limber up for a race. Science isn't much help for a definitive answer, as although the research does seem to suggest that post-running stretching can help to prevent injuries, it's by no means conclusive. With regards to pre-exercise static stretching, a number of studies have even shown it to have a negative impact on performance and increase the risk of injury. It's no wonder that runners are confused.

There does seem to be a growing consensus, though, that flexibility work as part of a balanced training programme is beneficial. Common sense and the fact that almost all elite athletes and coaches prescribe stretching is also a good indicator that it's something we should be doing. From personal experience I know that there are a number of niggles I'm prone to that I can keep on top of with some focused stretching work. With time so precious to all of us, knowing how, when and what kind of stretching to do to maximize its potential gains is key.

I've already mentioned top physio Tim Deykin, and he's got me up and running again after an injury on more than one occasion. Tim's CV is impressive, attaining his first Sports Science degree 30 years ago, and since then, having qualified as a physio, working with the British slalom canoeing squad, St Helen's rugby league team, and Olympic swimmers and cyclists, and being lead physio to the North West Institute of Sport. He also practises what he preaches, recently placing third in his age group in the European short course quadrathlon championships. By showing me how stretching is a key component of training, he has helped me conquer injuries and come back faster and stronger. I therefore took the opportunity to pick Tim's brain on this subject about how and why to stretch, and to get him to demonstrate an effective routine for runners. By understanding what you're doing, I hope it'll increase your motivation to make it a regular part of your training.

WHY STRETCH?

Rather than the usual vague 'to prevent injury', Tim has a 10-point checklist of reasons:

✓ The ability to hold sustained positions or postures, especially at the end of range of movement that normal activity may not cause. Working to these far ranges results in more flexible and functional tissue.

- ✓ Counteracting the effects of repeated movement patterns (such as running, cycling or swimming) that can develop muscle imbalances.
- ✓ Increasing range of movement, allowing for improvements in efficiency and economy of movement.
- ✓ Elimination of metabolites at end of activity.
- ✓ Elongation of muscles breaks tendency to develop trigger points (localized areas of tightness within a muscle).
- ✓ Development of trunk/core stability.
- ✓ Development of control, isolation and 'body awareness'.
- ✓ Learning to rise above pain, and how it can ease, does not always equate to injury in a state of mediation and relaxation.
- ✓ Counteracts stiffening effect of ageing on joints.
- ✓ Post-injury can help to reduce the formation of scar tissue.

WHEN TO STRETCH

Tim is adamant that the time to stretch is post-workout:

Stretches are best performed post-activity not only because the body parts are warmer and in a better thermal state for stretching, but because when muscle fibres are elongated, fluid exudes from between the fibres, where it can be transported away by the lymph system and circulation, so enhancing the removal of metabolites. In this sense the stretching routine at the end of a training session is not an add-on to the session you have just done. It should not be considered as being redundant with respect to the outcome of that session, as this will tend to give you the feeling that it is dispensable. You should think of it more as early preparation for the next session. Elongation of muscles, improved range of movement and the elimination of metabolites built up during strenuous activity all ensure an optimal muscle environment for your next workout.

Tim is the first to admit that stretching the moment you finish a run might not be realistic, and if you're cold and wet you might rush the job or not even bother. Get dry, get some warm kit on and then work through your stretches. It's not even the end of the world if you work through your stretches at the end of the day in front of the TV, just as long as you're doing them regularly.

HOW LONG TO HOLD EACH STRETCH

This is an area of controversy, but Tim is convinced that a stretch of one to five minutes is far more effective than the normally prescribed 15–30 seconds:

Holds of just 15 seconds have been reported to be enough to produce elongation in a muscle. However, it has also been demonstrated that with short duration stretches, the amount of elongation achieved is diminished when reassessed 10 minutes later to produce an overall lengthening of only 20 per cent of the stretch. Also, this seems far too short a period to overcome resistance to elongation by the very fact that a muscle is often painful when stretched, so it attempts to hold itself together, the opposite of elongation. Most importantly, every cell in your body is held in position by fascia, and this is a huge organ that can exist in two ends of a continuum between an immobile solid and a pliable gel. In both states it is composed of fibres embedded in a matrix (an aqueous mixture of chemicals). The fibres are what produce the tensile strength. The matrix can exist in a solid state or a gel state. Normally it is in the solid state, but it can transpose into the gel state under certain conditions such as mechanical factors such as movement, pressure or stretch, though this transposition is not instant and can take anywhere between two and five minutes to occur. This means that a short-acting 15-second stretch will not effect a change in this tissue. There has evolved a technique of soft tissue manipulation (specific deep massage) called myofascial release, and this employs deep pressure or stretch of a sustained nature to allow the fascia to transpose from the more solid to the gel (flowing) state. Sustained stretches not only allow us to access these elongation benefits, but on a neural level the initial resistance to stretch due to muscle tension can be painful or at least anxiety provoking, both of which reduce the benefits of the stretch, and generally there is a tightening of all the muscles around the affected part. Employing a sustained stretch allows you to relax the surrounding muscles during this phase and eventually to release the tension in the muscle you're stretching. If you continue to hold the stretch it seems as if you come to another level of relaxation and release, and so on in layers of relaxation and release. Eventually there is no pain or discomfort, and at that point you really feel like you are beginning to stretch tissues for the first time. No one can ignore this feeling of enlightenment.

THE ROUTINE

One of the first things you'll notice when you try this routine is that it's no soft option. It is a workout, you will sweat, but you'll really feel good afterwards. The routine below concentrates on the lower body and is great for runners. Aim to hold each stretch for a minimum of one minute, but if it feels really good, you've got the time, or the area feels especially tight, go for up to 5 minutes. In an ideal world you'd perform the full routine after every workout, but time constraints may prevent this. However, if you just go for a one-minute hold of each stretch, it only takes 12 minutes. Experiment with it and you'll find the stretches that are good for you, and you can concentrate more on those.

Indian knot

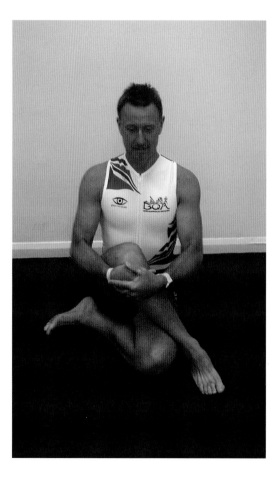

Indian knot

This is probably my favourite of all the stretches Tim has taught me and one that, much to my wife's consternation, I'll happily sit in front of the TV doing. Focusing on the buttocks and the sciatic nerve, it targets an area that is also often related to tightness in the hamstrings. Sit on the floor with one leg bent in front so the heel rests near the opposite buttock. Cross the other leg over, maintain a strong core and elongate through your spine. You should aim to distribute your weight evenly through both buttocks, although don't be surprised if one side is elevated. As you ease into the stretch it will even out. Hold for one to five minutes and then repeat the other way.

Lay-back

This is a real killer, but is probably the best quad stretch I've ever been shown. It'll also get into your hip flexors, ITBs and, if you do the full version, is a great core conditioner. Kneel down, brace your stomach muscles

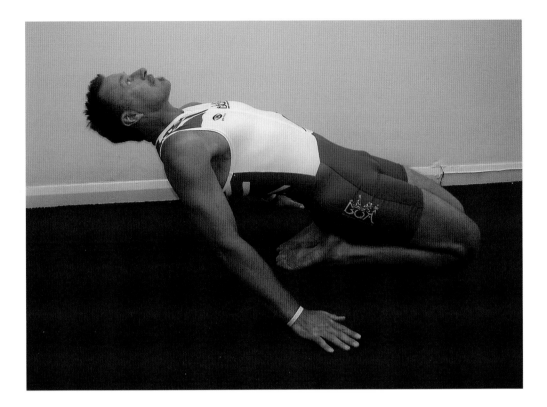

and lean back. Squeeze your knees together and engage your glutes to raise Lay back your hips. If you find this too much, use a chair to support your shoulders. Hold for one to five minutes.

Hamstring/psoas counter-strain

With this stretch, as you target the hamstrings on one leg the hip flexors on the other leg are stretching. The tightness of one muscle group provides a counter-strain to the other. Also, you're having to recruit all of your core muscles to maintain balance and good posture in this stretch. Begin by kneeling on one knee and then straighten the other leg out in front of you. Ease into the stretch by sliding the heel of the straight leg further away from you. Resist the temptation to open out your hips, and actively twist towards the extended leg to prevent this. Hold for one to five minutes and then repeat the other way.

Hamstring psoas counter

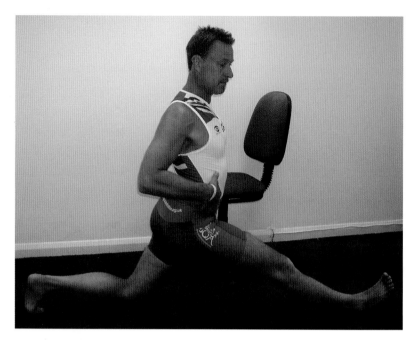

Gastrocnemius stretch

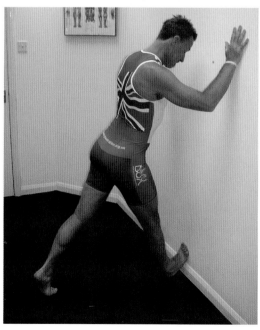

Calves

Gastrocnemius (upper calf). Place the foot of the leg to be stretched with the toes against a wall and the heel as near to the wall as possible. Roll the thigh outwards, tighten your quads and come up onto your toes on the other leg. Hold for one to five minutes and then repeat with the other leg.

Soleus (lower calf). Follow the same sequence as above, but push the knee of the leg being stretched towards the wall. Hold for one to five minutes and then repeat with the other leg.

Swiss ball crab

So many activities in training and daily life involve flexion of the lower back, so a whole body extension is a really good idea. Arch back over the Swiss ball and engage your buttocks to push your hips as high as possible. Hold for one to five minutes.

WARMING UP

Go to any race and you'll see people performing all sorts of bizarre warm-up routines. Bouncing, stretching, sprinting, jogging on the spot, you'll see them all, and knowing what you should do is confusing.

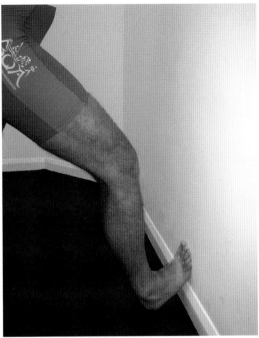

Soleus stretch

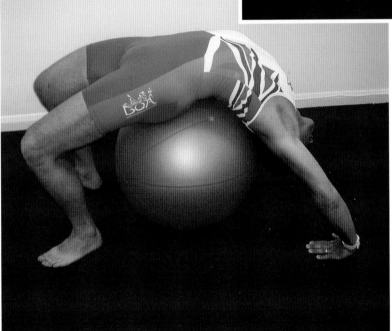

Swiss ball crab

The accepted rule is that the shorter the run, the longer the warm-up. This is why 100 m sprinters will warm up for ages and, because of the extremely explosive nature of their event, incorporate dynamic stretches and movements to prepare their bodies. For distance running, though, the only warm-up you need to do is to walk, jog and run for five to 10 minutes to loosen your body, raise your working temperature and get a bit of a sweat going. The overwhelming bulk of evidence indicates that stretching as part of a warm-up is not only totally ineffective but may actually reduce performance and increase the risk of injury. Also, if you stop to stretch after your warm-up jog, your body will just cool back down again.

Running Technique

You only have to watch an elite runner to appreciate the seemingly effortless grace as they float over the ground. Compare this with the plodding and shuffling hordes you see toiling round your local park. Both types of runners were born with the same innate ability to run, but the former, aided by genetics, great biomechanics and years of training, have developed, refined and hardwired their perfect running technique. For many people taking up running with the challenge of a marathon in mind, the last time they ran, apart from for the bus, would have been at school. Without having had years of regular practice and training, it's no wonder their running style leaves more than a bit to be desired. You never completely lose the ability to run, but that doesn't mean you're doing it well. The analogy I used in the introduction was someone attempting to swim the Channel without first making sure that their swimming technique was spot on. Swim miles in training using poor technique and you'll only get better at swimming badly. Bad habits become reinforced and you just make a tough challenge even tougher. The same applies to running. If from day one you overstride, plod heavily along, hunch up your shoulders and round your back and then continue to do so in training, you'll make those 26.2 miles an awful lot harder than they need to be.

Complete running novices almost have an advantage in this sense as they'll be starting from scratch and can develop their technique in tandem with their running fitness. Start off running well and you'll continue to do so. More experienced runners, who might have already even run a marathon, will have to go backwards before moving forwards. While they're undoing their old bad running habits, putting in long miles is a big no-no, as once fatigue kicks in so will the bad technique. Going back to basics and short runs where technique can be concentrated on is essential until the good new technique becomes second nature. I went through a similar process myself with swimming when starting triathlon. I could swim front crawl perfectly well and reasonably quickly, and had even swum at county level when at school. However, coming from a sprint swimming background, my technique was very much 'splash and dash', and although I could just about get away with it over sprint and Olympic distance triathlons (750 m and 1500 m swims respectively), stepping up to an Ironman distance race with its 3,860 m swim was out of the question. I went right back to square one and effectively relearnt to swim in an economical and efficient manner. It was deeply frustrating. I couldn't put in the hard swim sessions as my old bad form would re-emerge, and I was convinced my swim fitness was slipping away. I persevered though, and after eight weeks had a sleek new swimming stroke. Occasionally I still have to work through some drills to reinforce the techniques, but most of my bad old habits have disappeared, and my swimming is faster, more efficient and certainly less splashy. You can teach an old dog new tricks, and you can certainly teach an old runner to run better.

There are a number of schools and teaching philosophies dedicated to improving your running technique. These include Pose and Chi running, and many people have achieved great things by taking one of these courses. They are, however, very drill intensive and a big time commitment, and could involve you having to postpone your marathon plans while you master their techniques. A faster method to improve your running technique is to find a grassy field, kick off your shoes and run as nature intended, barefoot.

Now, before you start worrying that I'm going to get all hippy on you and start chanting, stick with me. I'm not proposing that you'll do all, or even a significant amount, of your running barefoot, but instead use it as a valuable teaching and training tool. Run barefoot and you'll run how nature intended: no slamming your heel into the ground, just a light, fast and more efficient forefoot strike. Try it: you'll instantly run lighter and faster. You'll strengthen and reawaken the muscles in your feet that have switched off and wasted from

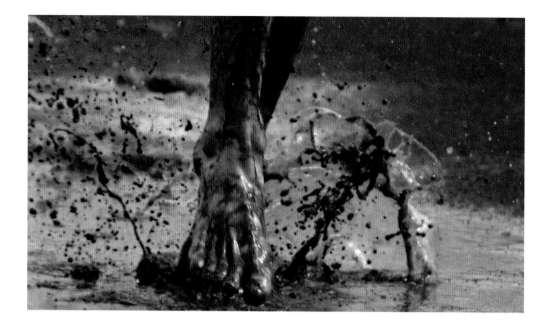

Barefooting: the fast way to perfect running technique

being entombed in shoes. Kicking off you shoes can be a fast-track way to a better running style and improved economy and speed. Many runners who've been plagued by injuries, such as plantar fasciitis, and have tried barefooting as a last resort, have found this more natural approach the cure to their ills.

The early stages of this plan, with short 20–30 minute sessions, are an ideal time to incorporate barefoot running. Don't feel as though you have to do all three sessions barefoot, but at least try to do one. As you run barefoot, focus on how your body feels from head to toe, and concentrate on these six coaching points:

Fast: Keep your cadence (foot-strike rate) high at 85–95 strikes per foot per minute. Check your cadence by counting the number of times one foot strikes in 30 seconds, and multiply the result by two.

Balance: Don't overstride, and avoid jamming your heel into the ground ahead of you. If you can see your feet in front of you, you're doing something wrong. Your feet should be under your centre of gravity and then lifted straight up under your hips at each stride.

Light: Think of yourself 'floating' over the ground and your feet lightly caressing the ground.

Tall: Stand tall and keep looking ahead. Don't hunch your shoulders, and keep your head up.

Relaxed: Keep relaxed, especially in the neck, shoulders and arms. Imagine you're holding a potato crisp between thumb and forefinger and can't break it.

Quiet: All of the above should lead to a quiet stride. Too much noise and something is wrong.

Keep working through these points in your mind, almost performing them as a body and technique scan as you run. Barefooting will reinforce what good running technique feels like, and then it's just a case of transferring those feelings to your shod running. When running with your shoes on, keep going through the checklist, and try to imagine the feelings your barefoot running evoked. With time, scanning your body and technique will become second nature, and you'll only need occasional barefoot sessions to remind you.

Walk to Run

One of the commonest mistakes novice runners make is just to go out for a run. Without the fitness, technique and pacing knowledge required, chances are it's going to be an unsuccessful, demotivating and painful experience. Four or five minutes in, you're bright red in the face, sweating profusely, your legs are burning, and your heart and lungs feel as though they're going to leap out of your chest. What chance have you of running for 26.2 miles if you can't even manage 10 minutes? For many people their 'running career' ends there and they join the ranks of people who mistakenly think they're just not runners. If you take a step back and think about it, though, is it really that much of a surprise that going out and running for 10 minutes solidly is beyond you? When was the last time you ran for any length of time? Maybe not since the horror of school cross-country. Even if you're reasonably sporty and take part in kick-abouts with your mates or the odd game of netball, the stop-start short distance sprints are very different from steady-paced continuous effort. Most people who are new to running expect too much too soon and try to run far too quickly.

Walking is something that, hopefully, if you're reading a book about running a marathon, you can already manage. You have the fitness to be able to walk continuously at a good pace and for a reasonable amount of time. You're able to judge your walking pace and effort to account for hills and to allow you to keep going. Walking is a genuine asset to the aspiring runner, and using it to develop your running makes perfect sense. By alternating walking and running you'll be able, from day one, to be out on your feet, moving with purpose and logging 10 minutes of running without experiencing the horror show we've just alluded to. As the workouts progress, your fitness and ability to judge pace and effort will improve and the proportion of running to walking will increase. After only eight weeks you'll be running strongly and comfortably for a full 30 minutes.

It's vital to get rid of the mindset that many runners have that walking is failing. It's part of the training plan and will get your to the goal of continuous running more quickly and less painfully than stubbornly trying to run no matter what. As a fell and ultra runner, walking plays a massive part in my own racing and training, and even the very top athletes in both disciplines use walk and run strategies. It's worth bearing in mind that a determined and fit walker can cover the 26.2 miles of a marathon in six to six and a half hours, which is quicker than many 'runners' manage. In fact, many marathoners who are taking five and a half hours or more would probably run a faster and more consistent race if, from the start, they alternated a minute of walking with a minute of running.

One of the main areas we're trying to develop by using a combination of walking and running is the skill and feeling of correct pacing. Most new runners try to run too fast too soon. This is often even worse in people who've come from a team sport where their default running pace is almost a sprint. It's vital to learn how to run economically, comfortably and at a pace that allows you to maintain that level of effort. It might feel painfully slow initially, but as you progress through the programme your steady pace will get quicker and, most importantly, it'll be sustainable.

The table opposite illustrates a 1–10 scale of self-perceived exertion that can be used to judge running pace and effort.

Score	Description/Feeling
1	Sitting on a sofa doing nothing
2	Getting up to make a cup of tea
3	Easy-paced strolling, none or slight feeling of exertion
4	Determined, purposeful walking. Having to concentrate, but still able to maintain a full uninterrupted conversation
5	Moving into a light jog, but still able to talk easily
6	Running 'Easy'. Still able to talk, feeling light, strong and comfortable
7	Running 'Moderately Hard'. Talking in limited to shorter sentences, starting to fight for breath, and really having to focus
8	Running 'Hard'. Single word answers only, and really starting to suffer
9	Running 'Really Hard'. Unable to communicate, and only sustainable for 10–30 seconds
10	Sprinting. 100% flat-out running … you're missing that bus

The level that we're looking to develop is Level 6 but many new runners who try to run continuously straight away rapidly find themselves creeping into Levels 7, 8 and even 9. The increments between the levels is really small, and without experience, staying in control of your effort is extremely difficult. Combining walking and running makes learning that control much easier.

As you do it day in and day out, finding your Level 4 determined walking pace shouldn't be at all hard. Scan your body as you walk, and note your breathing rate, how you feel and, most importantly, that you can maintain a full conversation. Having a training partner of a similar ability makes this much easier, as you'll be able to keep tabs on each other and make sure neither of you is pushing too hard. Ease into a run and be mindful of only letting your effort level rise slightly to Level 5 or 6. Keep talking, keep scanning your body, and think about the technique pointers we talked about earlier. For your first few running minutes you'll probably find you creep into Level 7, but you'll have a minute of walking to bring things back under control, and you'll know to rein things in a bit on the next running effort. After only a few sessions, you'll have found your running 'Easy' level (Level 6) and will have an effort level that'll see you all the way through to your marathon.

Running Shoes and Essential Kit

SHOES

It's essential that you start running in the correct shoes. Just digging out an old pair of plimsolls, trainers or gym shoes is a guaranteed recipe for injury. You don't have to spend a fortune on the latest super-supportive, ultra-cushioned and overengineered super-shoe, though. Many running shoe manufacturers and running shoe shops adopt a 'born broken' approach to running and gait, and by prescribing supportive shoes and even orthotics try to correct the faults they see in your running stride. There are two main problems behind this philosophy. First, if you're new to running and your body hasn't started adapting to it, there are bound to be faults with your stride, but rather than trying to correct them artificially, surely it's better to allow your training regime to make these corrections? Second, it's possible that the shoes might be *causing* the gait abnormalities. As we've already seen, running barefoot encourages an efficient, economical and sound running technique. If you keep support and cushioning to a minimum, re-creating that wonderful barefoot stride and allowing your feet to behave naturally is far easier. Because of the progressive approach of the programme, including focused strengthening work, the causes of poor and weak running will be worked on and corrected right from the start. This will negate the need for corrective shoes for the majority of people.

Start off buying a neutral, moderately cushioned shoe. I'm personally a big fan of Inov-8 shoes for running both on and off-road, and their Road-X 238 for women and Road-X 255 for men are ideal starting points. If you're already running regularly, entering the programme later on, and already have a favourite make and model of shoes that suit you, don't change a thing. However, if your running has been plagued by niggling injuries and you've been through different models of shoes and maybe orthotics without ever finding a lasting cure, seriously consider going back to square one, strengthen up, relearn to run and adopt a more minimalist approach to your footwear.

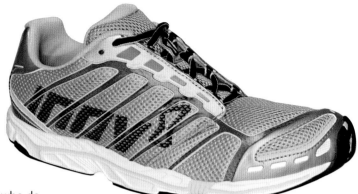

Typical road running shoe

There are obviously some people who do have anatomical features that need corrective intervention to allow injury-free running but, contrary to what the running shoe industry would have you believe, these people are in the minority. Follow the first eight weeks of the programme, and if after that you don't feel comfortable with your shoes, are feeling any unusual pain, or just don't feel right in your running, go to a specialist running shop and seek professional advice.

CLOTHING

That old cotton T-shirt and sagging leggings or baggy shorts aren't going to inspire you to get out and run, or do you any favours if you do try to run in them. Having proper running kit will not only give you the mental boost of looking and feeling like a real runner, but will make your running more comfortable and even easier. You're going to be investing a lot of time and effort into your running, so treat yourself to some decent kit.

SOCKS

As the interface between your feet and your shoes, the importance of good socks can't be emphasized enough. Wear the wrong socks and you could end up suffering from the curse of all runners, blisters. Different brands of socks suit different runners and different conditions, so it's really a case of trying a few until you find one that suits you. Look for a reasonable amount of padding and a material that wicks sweat and moisture away from your skin. Once you find a brand that works for you, buy enough pairs to see you through a week's running and replace them as soon as they start to wear.

BRA

For female runners, a properly fitted sports bra is as important as decent shoes. Get the fit or model wrong and you'll be distracted by straps falling off shoulders, painful movement and irritating chafing. Longer term you could risk tissue damage, causing your bust to sag. Seeking professional advice from a dedicated running shop is essential, and trying on a number of makes and styles is vital. Try to talk to running friends who are a similar size to you, and get their recommendations. What might suit the assistant in the running shop might not be suitable for you if you've got a bigger or smaller bust than her.

SHORTS/TIGHTS

There's no point in wearing big and baggy shorts to run in, you're just making life harder for yourself, and, if it rains, are setting yourself up for a truly miserable experience. Jogging and tracksuit bottoms are even worse and should be totally avoided. Running shorts need to be short enough to allow free movement of your legs and made of a fast-wicking/drying material. For guys, it's important they have a supportive liner to hold everything in place. If you're worried about chafing, or think you'd prefer more support, then a pair of cycling-style shorts can work really well. In colder weather, full length running tights are your best bet, and for those in-between spring and autumn days, Capri-length three-quarter tights are ideal. You can get different thicknesses of material, windproof and even fleece-lined running tights, so you should be able to find a pair for all conditions.

The Principle of Layering

With modern running kit there's no need to feel uncomfortable, cold or wet, no matter what the weather. In all but the most extreme conditions, your legs, as they're working, will stay warm with just one wicking layer on. If it's extremely cold and windy, light windproof leggings can be a good idea. On your upper body, though, a simple three-layer system allows you to control your temperature easily. With these three layers you'll be able to run in any conditions and easily adjust your clothing if the weather changes while you're out. You should always aim to start a run feeling slightly cold. If you start off

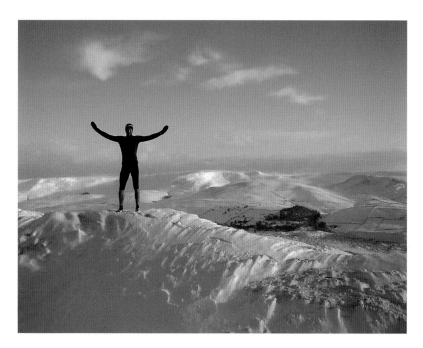

With the right kit and layers any day is a running day

warm and toasty, you'll rapidly overheat once you get going, and end up having to stop and remove layers.

BASE LAYER

Most important is the layer next to your skin. On many runs you'll just be wearing a single layer. A cotton T-shirt is just about the worse thing you can wear to run, and I always feel so sorry for charity runners who are obliged to wear the cotton T-shirts their charities have provided. Once you sweat, or if it rains, cotton just hangs on to moisture and keeps it next to your skin. This leads to chafing, bleeding nipples and, if the temperature's low, potentially dangerous chilling. A wicking base layer is designed to actively draw moisture away from the skin and onto the surface of the fabric, where it can evaporate. In hot weather this keeps you cool, and in the cold it makes sure you stay dry and warm. For warmer weather running, synthetic fabrics are hard to beat but, once the temperature drops, merino wool base layers are superb. Coming in a variety of thicknesses, cuts and styles, merino's wicking and insulating properties are the best even when completely soaked through.

MID-LAYER

Your mid-layer is an insulating layer that's there to keep you warm in cooler conditions. It should be loose enough to allow your base layer to function effectively, but not be baggy. That horrible old sweatshirt lurking in your wardrobe is not suitable. A mid-layer works by trapping a warm layer of air between it and the base layer and more warm air in its own fibres. It too should have wicking properties and can also be windproofed. Microfleece fabrics are ideal for mid-layers and give a high degree of insulation relative to their weight and bulk.

SHELL LAYER

Your shell layer protects you against the wind, rain and snow. On really cold days you might wear it over both your base and mid-layers, but for spring and summer showers it can go straight over your base. There are two main types of shell: windproof/water resistant; and waterproof. Windproof/water resistant shells tend to be lightweight, breathe really well, letting sweat and moisture out, and are relatively cheap. The downside is that although they'll give you some protection in the rain, anything more than a light shower will penetrate the fabric. This isn't too much of a problem on shorter training runs or on longer runs where you can easily find shelter, but if you're planning on heading out into the wilds or onto the hills for either a hike or a run, you'll want something more substantial. As its name implies, a waterproof should keep you totally dry, and to a certain extent they do. However, even though fabric technology has advanced substantially, a truly waterproof fabric that breathes well enough at genuinely high activity levels is still in the future. At the top end, the current crop of waterproof running jackets is good, but start pushing the pace and you'll be soaked through with sweat in no time. Expect to pay around £200 for a lightweight and breathable waterproof. This might seem a lot, but it should last a long time and it will be ideal for hiking and cycling too. Wholly urban runners will probably be better served by a quality windproof/water resistant shell, but for the more adventurous, a waterproof is a wise investment.

EXTREMITIES

Keeping your hands and head warm is essential for staying comfortable when running. With a hat and gloves you'll be able to wear less clothing and not have to worry about sweating heavily or overheating. You'll often see the elite runners at autumn marathons such as Chicago in shorts, singlets, hat and gloves. It may look at bit odd, but when you're running it really does work. On still winter days in temperatures as low as -5 °C, I'll head out in a base layer, shorts, hat and gloves. I'll be a bit chilly to start with, but after five minutes my temperature will be spot on. Another really useful bit of kit is a pair of cyclist's arm warmers. These removable Lycra sleeves with rubber stocking-style grippers at the top are brilliant for those in-between days when you can't decide between long and short sleeves. Hats aren't just for running in winter. A peaked cap for keeping the sun off your head and your eyes shaded in summer is vital for keeping your head cool and protecting you from possible heat exhaustion or sunstroke.

BUM BAG/RUCKSACK

Although for the first eight weeks of the plan your runs aren't long enough to necessitate carrying food or water, it's handy to have somewhere to stash your spare clothing layers, house keys and mobile phone. It makes sense, then, to sort yourself out with a

Rucksack

Bum bag

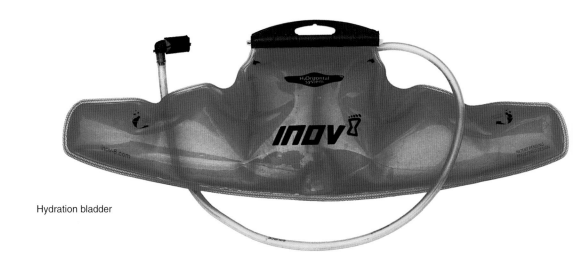

Hydration bladder

bum bag or small rucksack now. Look for one that gives you the option to carry a water bladder, or has pockets for water bottles. Make sure when loaded it's comfortable, doesn't bounce around, and has straps that allow you to compress it down when not full. Zipped pockets on the waist strap for easy on-the-go access to bars and gels are another key feature you should look for.

Cross-Training

Cross-training is using non-running activities as part of your running training. As with the strength training, many running manuals and marathon training plans skim over cross-training, relegate it to an activity for injured runners, and preach the outdated mindset of 'the only training for running is running'. This approach might work for elite athletes who have nothing to do but train, have full coaching, massage and physio support, and, when not training, can rest completely, but even they pick up injuries, and the more enlightened top level runners are now adopting a more varied and balanced approach to their training. For novices and any runners with the additional demands of work and family life, a cross-training approach to running is a far healthier, more moti-vating and more effective approach. In this plan, cross-training is an integral part of the programme and a key reason why you'll get to the start line fit, strong and injury free.

CYCLING

Cycling is probably the best complementary activity for runners. As well as developing your cardiovascular fitness and endurance, many of the muscle groups trained are the same as those used when running, especially the muscles you use when running uphill. Take a runner and put them on a bike and, although their heart and lungs will be up to the job, their legs will soon fail them. Take a cyclist and ask them to run and, although their legs will probably be sore the next day from the impact, their actual running performance will be pretty good. The reason for this is that the extra load of pushing a gear round recruits far more muscle than a running stride so, in simple terms, cycling gives you stronger legs. I can guarantee that you'll be extremely grateful for those strong legs when you're really having to dig in during the last few miles of your marathon. Cycling also has the benefit of being impact free, and provides a blessed relief from pounding the pavements. This combination of great fitness transferability to running and low injury risk make it the ideal cross-training tool. It's no coincidence that Ironman distance triathletes tend to bias their training massively in favour of cycling and, with proportionally little running, still manage to post sub three-hour marathon times even after an almost 4 km swim and 180 km bike ride.

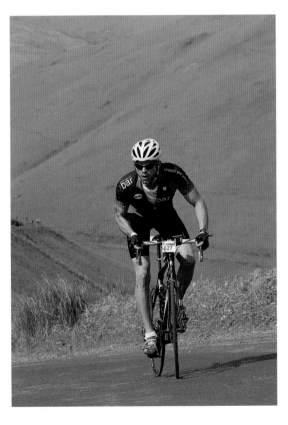

Nikalas Cook riding the 112-mile Fred Whitton Sportive in the Lake District

BUYING A BIKE

Most people have an old mountain bike lying around in their garage and, with a bit of TLC, a service at your local bike shop and, if you'll be riding on the roads, some slick tyres, you've got a perfect bike to start riding on. However, if you intend to follow the plan through to its end, getting hold of something slightly lighter, faster and more enjoyable to ride is a great idea.

Road bikes are typified by their curved dropped handlebars, light weight and skinny tyres. If all your riding is likely to be on the roads, this is probably the bike for you. Don't be intimidated by the racing looks. The handlebars offer a choice of three super-comfortable hand positions, and those skinny tyres make rolling along at speed a breeze. You'll also have a triathlon-ready bike should you want a new challenge after your marathon. Because of the growing popularity of Sportive or Challenge Rides (mass participation non-racing cycling events) there are now road bikes available with less aggressive non-racing geometry. This means your position will not be so low, but more comfortable and more suitable for recreational riders. The gearing on a sportive bike will also be far more suited to mortal riders, and a real bonus on hilly terrain. It's possible to spend £5,000 or more on a road bike, but a good alloy-framed bike with carbon forks and a decent spec can be bought for £400–£600.

Road bike

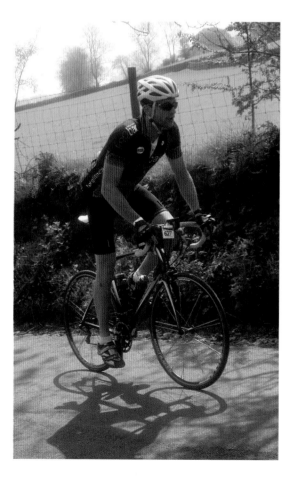

Mountain bikes are designed for tracks, trails and other off-road terrain. They'll be heavier than a road bike, have flat bars, front and possibly rear suspension, and much lower gearing. If you've got easy access to suitable trails, mountain biking is excellent fun and a brilliant all over workout. A good starting point for a basic hard-tail (front suspension only) bike is £400–£600, and £800 will get you a really good lightweight one. Unless you've got £1,200 or more to spend, don't be tempted by full suspension as you'll pay a massive weight penalty. You can easily put road-suitable tyres on a mountain bike, and many hard-tails allow you to lock out the suspension forks for more efficient on-road riding.

As their name suggests, hybrids sit in between road and mountain bikes. For some people they offer the best of both worlds, allowing efficient riding on the road as well as being suitable for light off-roading such as on canal towpaths. With flat bars they offer a more relaxed riding position, and some of the higher end models are surprisingly light and racy. The other side of the coin is that they're compromised by their versatility, and unless you live near a network of suitable bike trails you'd be better off getting one of the more specialized bike types. In my experience, most people who buy a hybrid usually end up buying either a dedicated road or mountain bike after a year or so.

Top of your additional kit list should be a helmet. Although not compulsory by law in the UK, helmets are so light and well ventilated now, there's really no reason not to wear one. Cycling shoes have a stiff sole that makes a massive difference to your pedalling. They also have cleats that, by a binding similar to those on skis, attach your feet to your pedals. Although this might sound scary, engaging and disengaging your feet becomes second nature in no time and 'being clipped in' facilitates a far more efficient pedal stroke. Cycling gloves, either fingerless mitts or full-fingered, not only protect your hands if you fall, but with anatomically placed padding, help to prevent numbness and discomfort in your hands. Sunglasses aren't just for posing and looking cool. A fly, piece of gravel or leaves on a low branch can really hurt when you're whizzing along, and even wind can make your eyes stream. Look for a pair with interchangeable lenses. You'll need dark/smoked for sunny days, red/orange/pink for overcast days, and clear for really dull days or riding at night.

One of the commonest problems

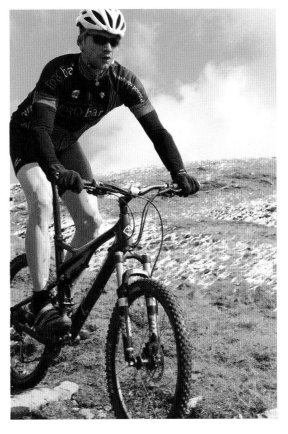

Mountain bike

people have with cycling is suffering from a sore backside. Don't make the mistake of going for a super-wide or heavily cushioned saddle, which will only make the problem worse. The solution is a quality pair of padded cycling shorts. Bib-style shorts with shoulder straps are best as they don't slip down and expose your lower back when you're leant forward on the bike. You'll also need a pump, spare inner tubes, tyre levers and a decent multi-tool. A good local bike shop will be able to advise you on kit, and some may also be happy to show you how to fix a puncture and perform basic get-you-home maintenance.

Spinning (or spin) classes can provide a fun and motivating way to get into cycling and build your riding confidence and fitness. Lasting 45 minutes to an hour, they're perfect for the cycling sessions in the first eight weeks of the plan, and will certainly add an intense edge to your training. Later on in the plan, as the rides increase to 90 minutes in length, you could always try doubling up classes, but there's no doubt that cycling for real outside is preferable. Riding a stationary spinning bike does little for your core stability, and you'll get so much more from riding outdoors. You'll also find, for the Sunday rides later in the plan, that the intensity of a spinning class will be too high.

No matter how much better cycling outside is for you, if you're training for a spring marathon through the worst of the winter, sometimes riding outside just isn't an option. Obviously, spinning classes or just an exercise bike at your gym are an option but, if you already own a bike, consider getting a turbo trainer. A turbo trainer is a small foldable frame that your bike is simply clamped to, transforming it into an indoor stationary trainer. The advantages of a turbo trainer are that you get to use your own bike that's set up correctly for you, it takes up less space than a traditional exercise bike, and is considerably less expensive. If your bike is a mountain bike you'll need to fit a smooth rear tyre. A fan to keep you cool also makes the experience more pleasant, and a few good DVDs or some motivating tunes will make the minutes pass faster.

During Level 1 you can ride however you want. If you're feeling strong you can push hard or do a spinning class, but if your legs are tired just ride on a flat course with an easy gear and spin your legs gently. Many people find this a far more effective recovery method than doing nothing. If riding indoors on a turbo or static bike, just dial the resistance right down.

In Level 2 the bike is there as a recovery session after your longer run. Resistance and gearing should be low and, if outdoors, your route should be as flat as possible. Really concentrate on maintaining a smooth, even and fast pedal stroke, and aim to keep cadence (the number of pedal rotations per minute) above 90 rpm. Fast legs doesn't mean hard, though, and you should imagine that your cranks are made of glass and that if you push too hard they'll snap.

For Levels 3 and 4 the bike still has a recovery element to it as it's non-impact, but we're also using it as a supplementary training activity to your long run. As your longest run will only be two and a half hours, compared with the three- to four-hour runs that many training plans prescribe, the cycling will make sure you build the necessary strength and endurance for your marathon without the injury risks that more running entails. The majority of the ride should be at a fairly easy pace, but there's no need to avoid hills, and you can push on if you're feeling strong.

SWIMMING

Swimming is an excellent cross-training activity for runners. As your body weight is supported by water, it's zero impact, and this makes it an excellent recovery session. You can still work your heart and lungs hard, get a great training effect and hit your upper body, but your legs have to do a minimal amount of work. The passing of the water over your muscles also has a therapeutic effect, and this will further enhance recovery.

Find out when your local pool or health club pool has lane sessions. Trying to do a structured and effective swim session while having to weave round children and inflatables is almost impossible. There will usually be a fast, medium and slow lane, so make sure you choose the correct one for your ability or for the stroke or drill you intend to do. If you find you're being over-taken regularly or are having to overtake, switch lanes. Also, don't obstruct the end of the lane when taking a rest, but make sure you move out of the way. If you're unsure of lane etiquette, ask the duty lifeguard.

If your swimming isn't up to scratch or you'd like to improve your stroke, look into taking a class. You'll still get the recovery and fitness benefits and will be learning a valuable new skill. Having been through the system, I can strongly recommend the Total Immersion method of swim coaching. It teaches a balanced position in the water and allows you to develop an economical and efficient stroke.

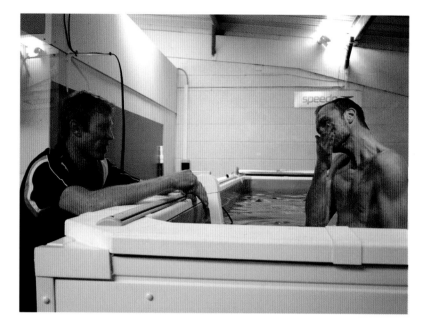

The author receiving swim technique coaching

Kit for swimming is minimal. If you're going to be swimming regularly, it's worth getting some racing-style trunks or a racing swimsuit. There's no point in slogging your guts out dragging a pair of baggy shorts through the water, or risking a potentially embarrassing accident during an overenthusiastic push-off wearing that old bikini. Proper trunks or swimsuits will offer the least possible resistance to the water, be cut to avoid chafing or rubbing and, as long as you rinse them well, be resistant to chlorine. Unless you have very short hair, a racing swimming cap will make you more streamlined and, if you have fair hair, will stop it taking on a green hue from regular exposure to chlorine. Goggles are important for protecting your eyes from the chlorine in the water and, most importantly, allowing you to avoid hitting other pool users and the wall at the end of your length. There are many different styles of goggles available, from the minimal unpadded ones that elite racers wear to more mask-style pairs that are good for open water swimming where a wider field of vision is advantageous. If you'll be swimming outdoors a lot, you might want a tinted pair with UV protection but untinted or lightly tinted ones are more suitable for indoor pool swimming. Anti-fogging is also a really useful feature to look for. When you go goggle shopping, try on a few pairs. Press the goggles firmly around your eyes without using the straps and, if the fit is good, they should stay put for a few seconds. Adjust the head strap so the goggles fit comfortably and stay put when you push off from the wall. Don't make it too tight, though, or it'll give you a headache. Finally, fine-tune the fit by adjusting the nose bridge. A pull-buoy is a float that you hold between your thighs, allowing you to concentrate on upper body form and to rest your legs. A kick-board is a float that you hold with your hands for doing legs-only drills. Hand paddles help to teach correct hand entry position into the water and, because of increased resistance through the water, make your upper body work harder. These last three bits of kit aren't essential, but incorporating them into swim sessions, such as the one described below, helps reduce the boredom of just ploughing up and down doing the same thing, and varies the training effect on your body.

This 30-minute swim session would be ideal for including in the plan:

0–5 minutes: Easy-paced swimming alternating front crawl, breaststroke and backstroke.

5–10 minutes: Hard front crawl lengths with 30-second recoveries.

10–15 minutes: Alternate two lengths arms only using pull-buoy with two lengths easy any stroke.

15–20 minutes: Alternate two lengths legs only using kick-board with two lengths easy any stroke.

20–25 minutes: Hard front crawl lengths, arms only, with pull-buoy and hand paddles. Recover for 30 seconds after each length.

25–30 minutes: Easy-paced swimming alternating front crawl, breaststroke and backstroke.

YOGA AND PILATES

Yoga and Pilates can both provide an ideal cross-training activity for the runner and can be great recovery day options. If you're lacking in flexibility or tend to be a bit unfocused with your stretching, a solid hour of supervised stretching in a yoga class can be really beneficial. Similarly Pilates, with its gentle but focused and controlled movements, is excellent for core strength and working those small but vitally important stabilizing muscles. Many running injuries can be traced back to these often neglected muscle groups.

I'd always been a bit of a yoga sceptic. Sitting around with crossed legs, chanting om and realigning my chakras wasn't really for me, and I was always convinced I'd be better off just going for another run or ride. However, attending a health and fitness retreat, including twice daily yoga classes, I was converted. For a very non-bendy runner and cyclist, the classes were extremely challenging, but two or three days into the retreat I felt as if I was making definite progress, and more importantly my running workouts felt super loose, fluid, relaxed and strong. I now have my own 10–20 minute yoga routine that I regularly work through, and whenever possible I'll join a class as a bit of a flexibility top-up. The other aspects of yoga that can be extremely beneficial for runners are the breathing and relaxation. The crossover of controlled breathing to running is obvious, and a relaxed runner tends to be a good and efficient runner. Learning to relax and breathe through stressful and uncomfortable poses transfers very well to holding your running form together in the final few miles of a marathon.

Yoga

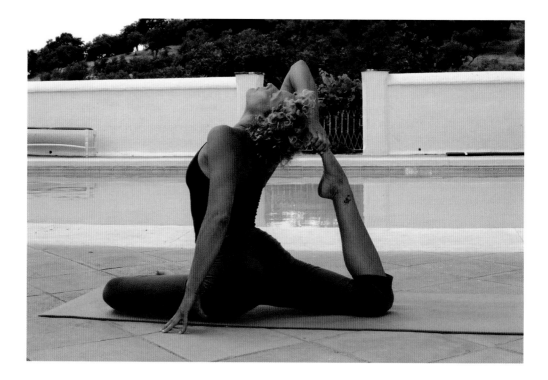

Yoga is an umbrella title for a range of forms, styles and approaches. It includes the extremely athletic and physically demanding Ashtanga or power yoga, Iyengar yoga with its props, straps and cushions, and even Bikram yoga, which takes place in specially heated rooms. Some classes stick to the physical side of practice, whereas other more spiritual ones might have you relaxing, meditating or even chanting. Many instructors fuse the different styles, so knowing which class to choose can be confusing. If you're going to a specialist yoga centre or trying to decide if a local class or class at your health club is for you, talk to the manager or the instructors and explain that you'll be practising yoga as a complementary activity to running. They should then be able to point you in the direction of a suitable class. Yoga classes often work in blocks so that everyone starts at the same level and works through learning the positions and sequences together. Try to find a fairly small class of 10 to 15 people, as individual attention from the instructor is vital. You'll think you've got a position right, and then the instructor will make a microscopic adjustment to you and it'll feel a whole lot different and usually a lot more painful. It's because of the precise nature of the positions, for both effectiveness and safety, that I'd strongly advise against the self-taught approach from a DVD or book. If you're keen to include yoga but unable to make a class, consider booking some one-to-one sessions. A good instructor will be able to tailor a routine to your individual needs and make sure you're doing things correctly.

Pilates is a training system that was developed in the early twentieth century by Joseph Pilates. He developed it primarily as a training and rehabilitation method for dancers, and that link to dance and dancers remains today. Pilates on its own won't give you that long and lean dancer's physique, but it is a good complementary activity to running. It emphasizes mindful control of the body to build strength, endurance and flexibility of the core muscles. Joseph Pilates referred to the core as the 'powerhouse' of the body, and although it's probably not the panacea of fitness that many Pilates enthusiasts and core-training evangelists claim it to be, there's no doubt that many of us could benefit from it. I came to Pilates after suffering from a lower back problem when cycling. The physio I saw happened also to be a Plilates instructor, and she used many of the classic exercises in my rehab. I now always include these exercises in my gym workouts, and my back is now stronger and pain free. As part of the mindful body control approach, Pilates, like yoga, places an emphasis on breathing techniques and relaxation. As with yoga, these aspects are directly applicable and beneficial to running.

The commonest and most accessible and affordable type of Pilates workouts are known as mat classes. Most gyms and health clubs offer these, although the quality and experience of the instructor and class can vary massively. Don't be afraid to ask about the instructor's qualifications, and speak to class regulars. As with yoga classes, because precision is essential for Pilates to be effective, look for smaller classes where the instructor can ensure you're performing the movements correctly. Without the correct instruction, focus and intensity, Pilates mat classes can be a bit of a nothing experience.

Although they're finding their way into general gyms and health clubs, Pilates reformer machines tend to be the preserve of specialist centres. Using a combination of springs, pulleys and your own body weight to create resistance, with the right instruction they can deliver a highly effective workout. Joseph Pilates developed his original reformers from modified hospital beds. Some larger centres offer classes on a fleet of reformers, but more commonly reformer work tends to be a one-to-one experience. This can make sessions very expensive, but if you decide that Pilates is for you and want to get the most out of it, investing in some personal sessions is probably the best approach.

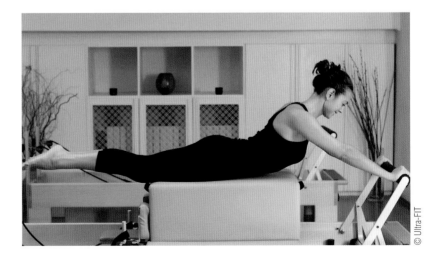

Pilates reformer

Hiking and Fast Packing

Once you've worked through Levels 1 and 2 of the plan and have built your running fitness and confidence to 10 km standard, getting off the roads occasionally and hitting the hills for your long weekend session can be a real boost to body and mind. Not only will you be lifted by the scenery and your surroundings, but you'll start to really appreciate the level of fitness you've attained and the possibilities this opens for you. A day on the hills will get you used to spending time on your feet and give you the confidence that you can manage a marathon. It'll also give you the chance to further experiment with your fuelling strategies.

For your hiking workouts you'll be adopting a fast and light approach. Rather than trudging away with a massive pack and heavy boots, you'll be using your running fitness and stripped down kit to cover the miles. When I think back to my school days, and specifically my Duke of Edinburgh expeditions, I shudder at the size of the packs we lugged round and the stiff, heavy and blister-inducing boots we rammed onto our feet. Even now, whenever I'm running on my local trails in the Peak District, or further afield in the Lakes or

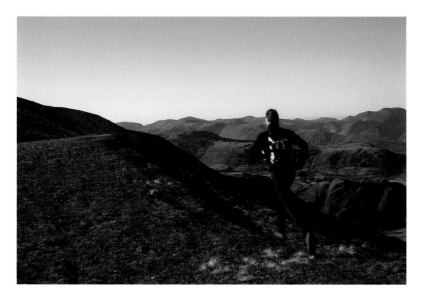

Fitness and fast packing open up the hills

North Wales, I still see people labouring under heavy packs, moving at a snail's pace with their gaze steadfastly fixed on the patch of ground immediately ahead. There's absolutely no need at all to make life so hard for yourself, and by packing light and moving fast you can extend your daily range, appreciate your surroundings more and massively increase your enjoyment.

Using the classic ultra-running pacing strategy of walking the climbs, jogging the flats and running the downs, you'll be amazed how much ground you can cover. Discipline in sticking to this pacing strategy is key for fast and light hiking success and is particularly important at the start of a day, when freshness and the freedom of the hills can cause you to overcook things. No matter how strong you feel, the moment the trail tilts upwards throttle back and shift to a purposeful walk.

Don't think that you have to head to genuine upland terrain such as the Scottish Highlands, Lake District, North Wales or my home patch of the Peak District. Any rolling countryside is ideal and will be a welcome change from pounding the pavements. It's important that the terrain is rolling, though, as otherwise you'll end up running too much and overdoing it. You need the hills to get the most out of these sessions and, odd as it may seem, to give your body a break from continuous running. Many areas of woodland managed by the Forestry Commission have ideal marked trails, and when I was based in London I regularly use to head to the Chilterns or North Downs.

If you're planning on heading to the hills, especially genuine upland terrain, then it's essential you're competent in the use of a map and compass. For lowland terrain and marked trails an Ordnance Survey 1:50,000 scale map is adequate, but for upland and mountainous routes the greater detail of 1:25,000 is essential. There's no point in moving fast if you're moving in completely the wrong direction. Being able to relate features on the map to the actual land, and vice versa, orientating the map to your compass and direction of travel, moving on a bearing in poor visibility, estimating distances, and being able to quickly plot your position and plan an escape route if conditions deteriorate are all essential skills. A GPS is a great piece of supplementary kit, but is no substitute for a map and compass. It's also vitally important to let someone know where you're planning on heading, and how long you expect to take. Carry a mobile phone, but don't rely on having any coverage in remoter areas.

It's also important that you have the right shoes for the job. Don't even think about heading off-road in your regular road shoes or you'll be spending a lot of time on your backside or even turning an ankle. Road shoes don't have enough grip for the mud, wet grass, loose gravel and rock you are likely to encounter. Also, because of the thicker cushioning road shoes tend to have, they hold your feet further off the ground, reducing stability and increasing the risk of a fall or a twisted ankle. Trail shoes have much more aggressive outsoles and less cushioning than road shoes and are designed to cope with the rough stuff. Again, Inov-8 offer a great range of suitable shoes.

No matter how benign the weather appears when you head out, it can change for the worse in a matter of minutes in the hills. Even in the summer you should carry a hat, gloves, a spare base or mid-layer, and a genuinely waterproof jacket. To carry this kit, as well as your water and food, you'll need a small (10–20 litre) day pack. Look for a pack that sits comfortably on your back and has straps that allow you to compress it down into a stable load. Other features to look for are zipped pockets on the waistband for easy access to snacks, a whistle integrated into the chest strap for signalling in an emergency, and the capacity and capability to carry a water bladder or bottles.

Hiking or trekking poles take a significant load off your knees and back and can make a massive difference to a long day in the hills. Setting the correct height of the poles is easy. With your arms by your sides, arms bent at 90 degrees and forearms parallel to the floor, the poles' grips should be level with your hands. The technique for using them when climbing is fairly obvious and should come naturally. There are a few key points to remember. Keep your head up and chest open. Don't overreach with the poles, keep them angled backwards and only place them a foot or so in front of you. On short downhills, just transfer the poles into one hand. For longer descents, break the poles down and stow them on the outside of your pack. For steep and technical downhills, poles can be a knee-saving joy.

The Plan

	Week 1	Week 2	Week 3	Week 4	Week 5	Week 6	Week 7	Week 8
Monday	Recovery session. Yoga/Pilates or rest	Recovery session. Yoga/Pilates or rest	Recovery session. Yoga/Pilates or rest	Recovery session. Yoga/Pilates or rest	Recovery session. Yoga/Pilates or rest	Recovery session. Yoga/Pilates or rest	Recovery session. Yoga/Pilates or rest	Recovery session. Yoga/pilates or rest
Tuesday	Run 1: 20 mins 1 min run/ 1 min walk Followed by strength routine	Run 1: 30 mins 1 min run/ 1 min walk Followed by strength routine	Run 1: 2 X 5 mins 1 minute walk reco Followed by strength routine	Run 1: 2 X 8 mins 1 minute walk reco Followed by strength routine	Run 1: 2 X 10 mins 1 minute walk reco Followed by strength routine	Run 1: 2 X 11 mins 1 minute walk reco Followed by strength routine	Run 1: 2 X 12 mins 1 minute walk reco Followed by strength routine	Run 1: 2 X 15 mins 1 minute walk reco Followed by strength routine
Wednesday	30 mins swim	30 mins swim	30 mins swim	30 mins swim	30 mins swim	30 mins swim	30 mins swim	30 mins swim
Thursday	Run 2: 20 mins 1 min run/ 1 min walk Followed by strength routine	Run 2: 30 mins 1 min run/ 1 min walk Followed by strength routine	Run 2: 2 X 5 mins 1 minute 1 walk reco Followed by strength routine	Run 2: 2 X 8 mins 1 minute 1 walk reco Followed by strength routine	Run 1: 2 X 10 mins 1 minute 1 walk reco Followed by strength routine	Run 1: 2 X 11 mins 1 minute 1 walk reco Followed by strength routine	Run 2: 2 X 12 mins 1 minute 1 walk reco Followed by strength routine	Run 2: 2 X 15 mins 1 minute 1 walk reco Followed by strength routine
Friday	40–60 mins cycle or spin class	40–60 mins cycle or spin class	40–60 mins cycle or spin class	40–60 mins cycle or spin class	40–60 mins cycle or spin class	40–60 mins cycle or spin class	40–60 mins cycle or spin class	40–60 mins cycle or spin class
Saturday	Rest day	Rest day	Rest day	Rest day	Rest day	Rest day	Rest day	Rest day
Sunday	Run 3: 20 mins 1 min run/ 1 min walk Followed by strength routine	Run 3: 30 mins 1 min run/ 1 min walk Followed by strength routine	Run 3: 30 mins 80 secs run 40 secs walk Followed by strength routine	Run 3: 30 mins 100 secs run 20 secs walk Followed by strength routine	Run 3: 30 mins 110 secs run 10 secs walk Followed by strength routine	Run 3: 30 mins 120 secs run 10 secs walk Followed by strength routine	Run 3: 30 mins 120 secs run 10 secs walk Followed by strength routine	5km Run or race Followed by strength routine

The Sessions

MONDAY

Monday is a recovery session or a complete rest day. A gentle yoga or Pilates class is an ideal option, or even a relaxing swim. Although you might be all fired up and enthusiastic about getting stuck into the plan, it's important to learn to listen to your body. If you feel at all tired, or your legs feel heavy, take a rest day. Think about getting a massage, or just work through some gentle stretches. Recovery is as important as training for gaining fitness.

TUESDAY

Alternating periods of walking and running, this session is where you start to learn the comfortable Level 6 'Easy Running' pace. Remember to continuously scan your body and think about your running technique. Even if these sessions feel too easy, stick with them and don't be tempted to skip ahead. A slow, gradual build-up and consistent training are essential. Rush through and you'll be trying to build your fitness on shaky foundations. The second part of the session is the strength routine. The walking and running work serves as the perfect warm-up, and it's impossible to exaggerate the importance of this strength work for your long-term running success. Don't be surprised if your legs are sore one to two days after your first few strength workouts. Known as Delayed Onset Muscle Soreness (DOMS), this is completely normal, shows that you have given your muscles a new training stimulus, and will ease.

WEDNESDAY

This is down as a swimming session and you'll find that some time spent in the water will have an almost miraculous restorative effect on your legs. Don't feel as though you have to swim hard: simply wallowing in the water will be beneficial. As with Monday, if you feel really tired, take a complete rest day.

THURSDAY

This is exactly the same as Tuesday.

FRIDAY

Friday is cycling day. Again, you have to listen to what your body is telling you. If your legs are tired and heavy, a really gentle flat ride or spin on a stationary bike against low resistance will really help them to recover. If you're feeling strong, or coming to running with a fitness base from other sports or training, a harder ride or a more demanding spinning class can be a great non-impact way to get a higher intensity training hit.

SATURDAY

No option, no choice: Saturday is rest day. Hopefully you'll be glad of the chance to put your feet up, but if you have one of those 'must do more' mindsets, rein in your enthusiasm and chill. Probably the biggest difference between full-time pro athletes and top amateurs is not the amount or intensity of training, but the recovery. Recovery is as big a part of their job as training. Spend time with elite pro athletes and, when not training, they're pathologically lazy. Their adage is, 'Why run when you can walk, why walk when you can sit and why sit when you can lie down?' I've never played so many video games or watched so many films as when I spent a week living and training with pro triathletes. Make the most of your rest time and see it as the key part of your training that it is.

SUNDAY

Another walk and run session, but with a slightly different focus from the Tuesday and Thursday sessions. As the plan progresses, the run intervals in this session don't exceed 120 seconds, but the walking breaks come right down to 10 seconds and eventually zero. You'll be applying the pacing and the Level 6 'Easy Running' that you've learnt in the Tuesday and Thursday sessions, and the shorter walks should just break up the session and provide you with enough time to scan your body and technique and compose yourself. If you're having to catch your breath, you're pushing too hard on the runs. This session is followed by your third strength workout of the week. The three strength sessions are essential for building those rock solid running fitness foundations, and although you'll drop to two and eventually one per week they're a consistent and essential part of the plan. The strength work you put in now will bullet-proof you against injury as your running volume increases and you progress towards your marathon goal.

CHAPTER 2

Level 2: Weeks 9–12

Introduction

Congratulations on making it through the first eight weeks of the plan and on becoming a runner. Getting through the first block to running 5 km from a non-running start is probably the hardest part of the entire plan. You should now, with the progressive approach to running, key strength workouts and cross-training sessions, have found your comfortable running pace and feel as though your confidence and running ability are rapidly increasing.

The next block, although doubling the distance to 10 km, is only four weeks long. Don't panic and think that this is too big an ask, you've already got enough strength and fitness to run 10 km if someone forced you to, and although it may seem hard to believe, the physiological difference between running 10 km and running 5 km isn't that great. This block is all about consolidating your gains, introducing some new training ideas, and keeping your running fitness moving steadily forwards. You'll also probably notice a genuine sense of a real leap forward in your fitness during this block. After 10–12 weeks of consistent training, significant and noticeable physiological changes will take place in your body. Muscles will have become stronger and the engine of your heart and lungs will have become more efficient. Enjoy the change, enjoy feeling strong, but don't get carried away. Stick to the plan, don't be tempted to skip ahead, and you'll soon have 10 km ticked off.

Hydration on the Go

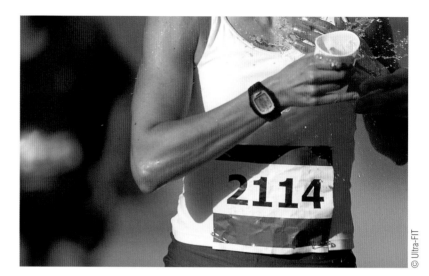

Keeping hydrated is essential for running success

With runs now moving into 30–60 minutes duration, it's time to start getting used to drinking on the go. Although it's perfectly possible to run for longer than this without taking fluids on board, it'll pay to start getting use to sipping on the move, and experimenting with drinks and drinking systems before it becomes essential. Up to 80 per cent of your body is water. Studies have shown that as little as a two per cent drop in body weight through dehydration can affect exercise performance. A loss of five per cent can decrease the capacity for work by up to 30 per cent. Many people who think they've hit the legendary Wall during a marathon have in fact simply let themselves become dehydrated. There are a number of reasons for this drop in performance:

✓ Reduction in blood volume.
✓ Decreased skin blood flow.
✓ Decreased sweat rate.
✓ Decreased heat dissipation.
✓ Increased core temperature.
✓ Increased rate of muscle glycogen (the body's energy store) use.

Once your body has started down the slippery slope of dehydration, it's very hard to rescue the situation, and if you continue to try to push on and keep running you'll only get slower and slower and run the risk of heatstroke. Waiting until you feel thirsty before drinking is too late, as once your body is telling you you're thirsty your performance will already be compromised. Ensuring that you're adequately hydrated before running, and then adopting a little and often approach to drinking right from the start of a run, is the only way to ensure that dehydration doesn't slow you down.

One of the main reasons for runners, especially female runners, not drinking adequately is worrying about not being able to find a toilet or, in a race, losing valuable minutes taking a pee stop. With practice and experience, though, it's possible to find a rate of fluid intake that keeps you hydrated but doesn't leave you constantly needing the loo. Finding this rate, which will be personal to you, is another reason for practising drinking from this early stage. Plan your training routes to include a couple of potential pee stops just in case, and in a race you'll lose less time having a Portaloo moment than if you let yourself become dehydrated.

Knowing how much to drink is a personal thing, and finding your optimal intake is a matter of trial and error. It's also affected by climatic conditions and by how hard you're working. Some coaches and running guides recommend weighing yourself before and after runs to find out how much water weight you're losing, but personally I think this is complicating the issue. From personal experience I've found that, for an average sized male runner (75 kg), an intake of 500–750 ml per hour is about right. A smaller (50 kg) runner might only need 250–500 ml per hour. The key to optimal running hydration is not to get hung up on total amounts, though, but instead to stick religiously to the 'little and often' mantra. Taking a sip every two to five minutes right from the start of your run is the winning habit to get into. After a few runs of trying this, you'll soon find a rate that works for you, doesn't have you constantly searching for a loo, and soon becomes second nature. Getting this habit ingrained is absolutely vital to running and marathon success, and if you find you struggle to remember to keep sipping, set an alarm on your watch to remind you.

For runs of up to 60–90 minutes, and for getting used to drinking on the run, plain water is perfectly adequate. However, your body has a variety of salts and minerals dissolved in its fluids that are vital to it functioning. Diluting these too much with excessive consumption of plain water can be as detrimental as allowing your body to dehydrate. As runs get longer, not replacing these electrolyte salts can lead to cramps, muscle failure and, in extreme cases, collapse. Fortunately you can buy effervescent tablets such as Nuun that, when dropped into a bottle of water, deliver the perfect balance of electrolyte salts. They also have the advantage of adding some flavour to the water, which makes you far more likely to drink it. There's no harm in experimenting with different brands and flavours at this stage in the plan and finding one that suits you now.

As well as delivering electrolyte salts, it's also possible to use your fluid intake to deliver some of the calories you'll need for longer runs. This isn't really an issue at this stage of the plan, and we'll talk more about sports drinks when we deal with fuelling longer runs later in the plan. At this stage it's probably best to avoid these energy drinks. You won't need the additional calories they provide for the length of runs you'll be doing, they'll be counter-productive if you're wanting to shed a bit of weight, and by providing sugar for your body to burn you'll be compromising your body's ability to burn fat as a fuel.

As with most aspects of running, what drinking system suits you is down to personal preference. Some people love the feeling of a bottle in their hand and find it hard to run without one. Others find that it throws them off balance and prefer a bum bag to hold their bottles, or even a fluid bladder. Again, it comes down to experimentation, and now's as good a time as any to start experimenting. As well as standard cycling bottles, it's possible to get bottles with a strap that goes around the back of your hand. If you don't mind the feel of a bottle in your hand, then these, along with 'doughnut' style bottles with a hole in the middle, can be ideal for shorter runs or longer runs or races where you have the opportunity to refill. There are a number of bum bags and rucksacks that have holsters for one or two bottles. Although this is probably overkill at this stage in the plan, if you can find one that suits you now it'll serve you through to marathon day. You want to make sure it doesn't bounce excessively or rub, and that the bottles are easily accessible while running. The final option is a bladder with a drinking tube that sits within a bum bag or backpack. Known as hydration packs, if you can find one you get on with they make drinking on the go super easy, and, if drinking is easy you're more likely to do it. The drinking tube will have a bite valve on it that allows for hands-free drinking, and bladders ranging in size from one to three litres are available. You obviously don't have to completely fill the bladder if you're doing a shorter run, and by inverting the bladder and sucking the air out you can prevent it sloshing around annoyingly.

Music on the Run

With MP3 players, having some motivating tunes to accompany you on your runs has never been easier. I remember the dark old days of Walkman cassette players and supposedly portable CD players that'd skip and jump at anything more vigorous than a gentle stroll. There are a number of factors to consider, though, before deciding whether to use music during your training.

The effect of music on exercise performance has been extensively studied, and there have been some extremely positive findings for aspiring marathon runners. One of the key effects that listening to music can have is to narrow your attention and divert the mind away from the sensations of fatigue. This is known by psychologists as dissociation, and because of it your perception of effort is reduced. Music can raise your mood and enhance feelings of wellbeing such as vigour and happiness. Conversely it lowers negative feelings such as tension, depression and anger. A happy, relaxed runner is always going to outperform a miserable uptight runner. These effects have been shown to be especially significant at low to moderate exercise intensities and therefore very relevant to steady-state distance running. At these intensities, studies on treadmill running have shown an up to 10 per cent reduction in perceived exertion when running with music. As exercise intensity ramps up and sensations such as burning muscles and shortness of breath increase, the effort-masking effect of music decreases. However, the mood-enhancing effects remain, making the workout considerably more enjoyable. The music won't necessarily help with *what* you feel at higher intensities, but it will certainly help *how* you feel. These dissociative and mood-enhancing effects would seem to make plug-ging in your headphones a no-brainer, but there are downsides. Particularly during the early stages of the training plan I want you to be really aware of how you're feeling when you're running, and concentrating on finding your steady-state, comfortable running pace. The dissociative powers of music will inhibit your doing this, and zoning out can easily lull you into running too fast. On race day, do you really want to be dissociated from the experience? The crowds lining the route of a big city centre event and the support and camaraderie from fellow runners during any race can be a far bigger boost and distraction to your fatigue than even your favourite tunes. Your time spent running can also be the one time during the day when you're switched off from modern life, have some head space, and can take the time to truly appreciate your surroundings. Do you really want to be dissociated from that? Personally, especially when I'm running out on the hills, the sounds of nature are better than any music.

Music can have a massive effect on your running pace and rhythm. You can't help but match the beat of the music with your foot strike. This can be incredibly positive. Haile Gebrselassie would train to 'Scatman' prior to world record attempts as he found that the tempo matched his target strike rate perfectly. For a hard interval session or tempo run, choosing tracks that match your pace can make a real difference to the quality of a session. However, for longer runs where you're trying to develop your comfortable pace, the beat of music can easily cause you to vary your pace, run too hard and not achieve the workout's objectives. If you find you must have some distraction on longer training runs, try some podcasts or audiobooks. There are some great running podcasts and, as I did when putting in training runs of eight hours plus for an Arctic ultra, catching up on some classic books gives you the bonus of some cerebral development.

There are also safety concerns to running with music. It certainly makes you less aware of traffic, which can be hazardous in both urban environments and on rural lanes and roads. Although attacks on lone female runners are extremely rare – and I'm loath even to bring the topic up – they do happen, and not being able to hear someone approaching from behind definitely puts you at greater risk. There are earphones available that are designed to not completely cut you off from the outside world, and you can always just have your music playing into one ear. As regards races, I was fully behind the organizers of the New York marathon's 2007 decision to completely ban earphones and personal music players. There's no way you can hear and respond to other runners who may want to overtake you, or hear important information that race marshals may be trying to pass on to you. I remember taking part in an off-road duathlon (run-mountain bike-run) that used the same loop for the run and the bike. I was amazed when I was on the bike and passing a number of runners who were wearing earphones and so were completely oblivious to me careering up behind them at high speed. Along with several others, I complained to the race organizer, and he banned personal music players the next year. I firmly believe that this should be the case in all races. This is a further reason for not becoming too reliant on music during training. If you do all your training with music and then find you're not allowed to listen to it on race day it could have a significant impact on your performance.

Weighing up the pros and the cons and, based on personal experience, I'd recommend the following guidelines for music on the run:

✓ For all runs in Level 1, when you should be really focusing on finding your running form and pace, and for all LSD (long steady distance) runs in the rest of the training plan, when consistent pacing is everything, I'd recommend not using music. If you find you need some form of distraction for these longer runs, go for an audiobook or podcast, but remember, you might not be allowed it on race day. Even if you know music will be allowed, don't become totally reliant on it. You don't want a flat battery or a failing MP3 player knocking your confidence on marathon day.

✓ If music is allowed on race day and you really feel you need it, be considerate of other runners and don't have the volume so loud that you can't hear anyone. I'd strongly recommend having your player with you but only plugging into it when you really need it. I know plenty of music-driven runners who've successfully used the crowd and race day atmosphere to get them through the first 18–20 miles of a marathon and then plugged into their special motivating playlist for the last six to eight miles when the going got really tough.

✓ For any runs where there is likely to be traffic passing near to you, at dawn, dusk or in the dark, or if you're a lone female runner, seriously consider the safety implications of running with earphones.

✓ Music can be a real lift during higher paced tempo and interval sessions. Experiment to find tracks that match your required speed, and even create playlists of alternating fast and slow tempo tracks for interval sessions.

Running Buddy

The best running companion you can have

Although there's no doubting that sometimes there's nothing to beat the peace, solitude and freedom of running on your own, there are a massive number of advantages to having a few reliable running buddies.

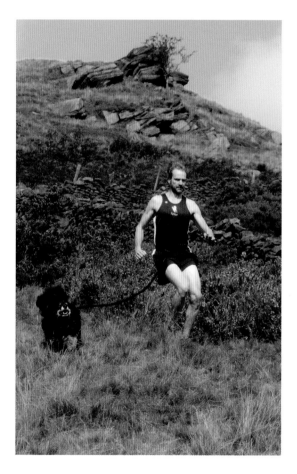

If you're starting the plan from square one, having a friend going through the process with you can make a real difference. You'll have someone to share your highs and lows with, and you'll be able to encourage each other and make sure that neither of you is slacking or skipping sessions. Early on, when you're finding your comfortable running pace, being able to chat to a running companion is the best indicator that you're not pushing too hard. Even as you become more experienced, on longer runs the 'chat test' is still hard to beat for correct pacing. You'll also find, especially if you're having to train either early in the morning or late at night, that getting started is the hardest bit of the session. Knowing you've arranged to meet a friend and not wanting to let them down can be a real boost to getting you out of the door. For faster paced sessions, there's no harm in a bit of low-key competition to help raise the intensity, and from a safety perspective running in a pair or a group is definitely preferable.

The next stage from running with a friend or group of friends is to join a local running club. Too many novices make the mistake of thinking you already have to be a great runner before you can even consider joining a club. In reality, novices probably have the most to gain from joining a club, and in most clubs they are brilliantly catered for and made to feel extremely welcome. As well as organized club training sessions, you'll find runners of your level who you'll be able to train with, you'll receive valuable tips from experienced runners, and you'll be able to find out about races that fit into your training programme. To find out about your nearest club go to *http://www.uka.org.uk/grassroots/search/*.

The biggest potential downside to training with other runners is that their pace may not suit you. It's vitally important for the success of the plan that you stick religiously to the paces and intensities specified, and that they are personal to you. It's perfectly possible, especially if you're starting from the same point, that your running buddy will progress at the same rate as you, but if at any stage you find yourself being dragged along too fast, or slowed down, it's better for both of you to look for a new partner. I've seen too many people stick with running partners – even making a pact to stay together on marathon day – out of a misplaced sense of loyalty, and ruining both of their runs. Being a member of a club, or having a group of running friends, is much better than relying on one partner. You should always be able to find someone who is currently at your pace or level, and you won't be left in the lurch if your partner picks up an injury.

The final aspect of club running to be aware of is that many of the coaches and more experienced runners at running clubs will be dyed- in-the-wool old school in their approach. They might well scoff at you approaching running from a cross-training perspective, and will argue that the only training for running is running. Stick to your guns, though, stick to the plan and maybe, once they see your marathon success, you might change their minds.

Get Off-Road

Although the majority of you will be training for a road marathon, I'd strongly recommend, whenever possible, getting off the road and hitting the trails. Some coaches and runners will say that you have to get your legs used to the pounding of the road, but I'd counter that the benefits of off-road running far outweigh any supposed impact resistance that hours of tarmac pounding will give you. Mud, grass and sand will force you to work harder, delivering an unbeatable running-specific strength workout and supercharging your legs. Hills tend to be more commonplace and significantly steeper than you'll encounter on the road, again raising the intensity of the workout. Slippery surfaces mean that you'll be working your core stabilizer muscles that are able to just switch off when you're on the streets. Technical terrain such as roots and rocks will literally keep you on your toes, encouraging a more efficient forefoot-striking running technique and a fast and light cadence. All of this will translate into stronger, faster and more efficient running when you do return to the roads. Along with all the performance benefits that off-road running can confer, it'll also make you happier and healthier. You'll be away from fume-spewing traffic and, without wanting to come over all tree hugger, getting back in touch with nature will give you a real mental lift. The joy of being on the hills on a clear, crisp and frosty morning is hard to beat, and the childlike pleasure of getting absolutely covered in mud never loses its thrill. You'll be less prone to overuse injuries, as every foot strike is completely different, unlike the repetitive thud of road running.

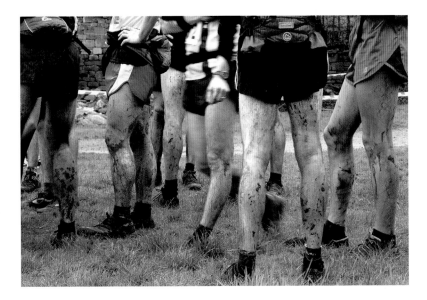

Fell running tools of
the trade

Off-road running doesn't have to mean extreme terrain and killer hills. Many disused railway lines have been converted to great running and biking trails, parks often have marked running routes, and many areas of Forestry Commission land have designated trails. It always used to amaze me when I lived in London and regularly used to run in Richmond Park how many people would mindlessly trudge around the outer loop unaware of the wonderful trails that criss-crossed the centre of the park, offering views of beautiful heathland, herds of deer and spectacular lakes, and a genuine escape from the panting masses.

Coming into Level 2, with a good base of running strength and fitness in the bank, is the perfect time to introduce some off-road runs into your training. Your LSD run at the weekend is ideal for off-roading. Look for undulating or rolling rather than genuinely hilly terrain, and if there are any significant hills don't worry about having to walk to maintain the correct exertion level. You'll soon find you'll be able to run those hills while maintaining the same level of effort. The following tips will help.

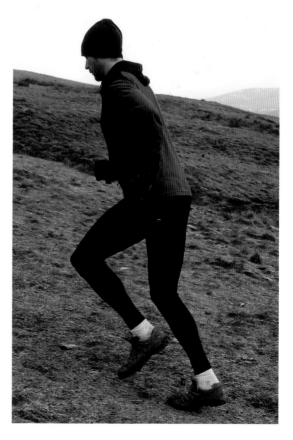

Good uphill technique

RUNNING UPHILL

The only way to build climbing strength is to simply get out and practise it. Learning to pace climbs, so you don't blow before the top, takes practice and a good fitness base. Having good hill strength is a big bonus in any runner's armoury.

Gear down: Like shifting down gears on a bike, as the terrain gets steeper shorten your stride. If you think you need to take two steps, take three. Keep light and up on your toes and the balls of your feet, and pump your arms.

Vary your angle of lean: The more you lean forwards, the more you bring in your powerful buttock muscles. Lean too far forward, however, and you'll upset your balance and restrict your breathing. Find a happy medium for the slope you're climbing.

Walk: Walking isn't admitting defeat, but is a significant part of off-road running, even for top fell runners. Purposeful uphill walking is often faster and more energy efficient than running as the gradient kicks up. When it gets really steep, pushing down with your hands just above your knees really helps.

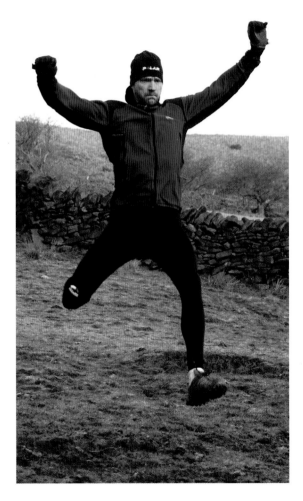

Letting it rip heading downhill

RUNNING DOWNHILL

What goes up must come down. Descending fitness and skills are as important, if not more so, than climbing strength. Again, it boils down to practice and training, but take it easy to start with or you'll be nursing sore legs for days.

Balance: Stay relaxed and use your arms to aid balance. Use body lean as your brake and accelerator. Lean forwards to speed up, and back to slow down.

Foot plant: The temptation is to lean right back and jam your heel in, but this is a guaranteed recipe for a tumble (scree slopes and deep snow are exceptions). Flex your foot down so that as much of your sole as possible makes contact with the ground and maximizes grip.

Line choice: Just like skiing or mountain biking, picking the right line is essential. Look ahead, and scan continuously for hazards or faster options. Don't just follow the herd: sometimes deviating off the beaten track can be faster and smoother.

Although there is a higher risk of acute injuries such as twisted ankles, this can be greatly reduced by using appropriate footwear. You'd be amazed how many people try off-road running in their heavily cushioned and grip-free road shoes, and are put off by the slipperiness and lack of stability. You wouldn't drive a road car off-road, so why try the same with running? True off-road running shoes are stripped down and lightweight with super-aggressive soles. Your foot is held close to the ground to maximize stability and prevent those ankle rolls; low levels of cushioning let your foot 'feel' the trail, giving crucial traction and directional feedback; and a soft, studded, sticky rubber sole grips no matter how filthy the conditions underfoot.

If you are running in a remoter location than a local park, it's important to carry a few bits of kit. A hat, gloves and a waterproof jacket with a hood weigh next to nothing and can be life-savers. An energy bar or a few jelly babies will keep you moving if you're out longer than you expected, and a foil space blanket will keep you warm and protected from the wind if you have a problem. Always carry a whistle to signal for help if need be, and if you're in an area you don't know, then having and being able to use a map and compass is essential. It's also a good idea to carry a mobile phone, although don't rely on having a signal. All of this kit can easily be carried in a bum bag or small rucksack. Finally, let someone know where you're planning on going and how long you intend to be out for. Obviously, running with a group or a running partner is preferable, but you should still carry suitable kit for yourself.

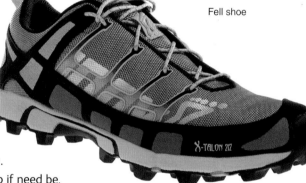

Fell shoe

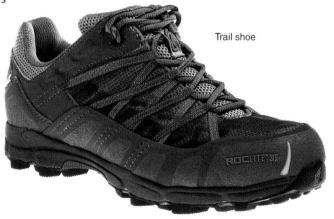

Trail shoe

The most important piece of kit for fun and success off-road is a pair of specialist shoes. A trail shoe sits in between a road shoe and a full-on fell shoe and is designed to cope with mixed rough terrain as well as running on hard-packed trails or even on roads. If you're planning on really heading off the beaten track, you might want to consider a fell shoe. Best described as a slipper with 4 x 4 capabilities, a fell shoe will have the following features:

1) **Upper**: Minimal, lightweight and quick drying. Some shoes at the 'trail' end of the spectrum will have waterproofing, but the usual philosophy is that mud and water will get in, so let's get it out as quickly as possible.
2) **Mid-sole**: Little or no cushioning keeps the foot close to the ground for stability. Flexible to allow the foot to behave naturally, adapt to the ground and maximize traction.
3) **Sole**: Aggressively studded, grippy rubber to give confidence when climbing, descending or contouring on a variety of surfaces.

If the off-road bug bites, and as your running fitness and confidence increase, you might like to try some off-road racing. Off-road racing can roughly be divided into three types:

Cross-country: Short, sharp blasts through the winter over parkland terrain. Races are typically 3–8 km, and although there are often some climbs and mud the courses are usually non-technical and conducive to fast racing. Most racers will wear cross-country specific spikes, but lightweight fell shoes are becoming popular, especially in junior races. The best way to get into cross-country is to join and race with a local athletics club. Go to *www.uka.org.uk* to find a club near you.

Trail running: Sticking to trails, footpaths and bridleways, trail races range from beginner-friendly 5–10 km events to full on 100-mile ultras. No navigational skills are needed as the courses are always clearly marked. Conditions underfoot will vary massively, and on some of the more extreme courses don't be surprised to find yourself doing a bit of wading. Go to *www.trailrunning.co.uk*, *www.humanrace.co.uk* and *www.trailplus.com* for information and events.

Fell running: A hill, fell or mountain is chosen, and you just race up and down it. Sometimes a series of climbs are linked together for longer races, but you still always have the same combination of hellish lung-busting climbs and exhilarating leg-sapping descents. Races vary from short, up and down 5 km blasts to two-day mountain marathons. Roads are avoided at all costs, and footpaths only used if strictly necessary. In a single race you may have to deal with rocks, mud, heather, peatbogs, grass, and even streams. Routes usually aren't way-marked, so you need good navigational skills, and as the taking of short cuts is encouraged, local knowledge is a distinct advantage. Go to *www.fellrunner.org.uk* for information.

Common Injuries: Avoiding and Treating

If you follow the plan to the letter, stick to the prescribed intensities and durations of workouts, don't skip ahead or miss sessions, and are diligent with your strengthening and stretching work, you should only need to read this section out of interest rather than necessity. I was in two minds about even writing a section on injury as I'm confident that if you follow the plan from start to finish then you'll run an injury free marathon. Runners will jokingly say that they're either injured, recovering from an injury or just about to get injured, and if you take a look at any of the runners' forums on-line this certainly appears to be the case. I firmly believe that this doesn't have to be so and that, with the correct foundations in strength and technique and a less tunnel-visioned approach to training, running can be an injury free activity.

TYPES OF RUNNING INJURIES

Running injuries can broadly be distinguished into two types: acute, and chronic overuse.

Acute injuries are sudden traumas such as a twisted ankle, a bruised knee from a tumble, or even being thwacked in the eye by a low-hanging branch. They're all freak accidents that happen entirely by chance, and if you're unlucky enough to suffer one you just have to accept the recovery time, find what activities and training you can manage, and seek professional advice as to the optimum and quickest way to get back running. Immediate treatment for the most common acute running injury, the twisted ankle, is described on page 73.

Chronic overuse injuries are the classic niggles, pains and debilitating conditions that plague runners. Most can be traced back to soft tissue, muscles, tendons and ligaments, weaknesses, imbalances or tightness. In most cases the actual running isn't the problem; it's trying to run with a body functionally compromised by hour upon hour of sitting. With the strengthening and stretching work, we're undoing the damage of sitting, and turning you back into a fully functioning running machine. Another classic cause is simply over-doing the mileage. Using a cross-training approach and not obsessing about three hour-plus runs reduces the mileage strain on your body and significantly reduces your risk of injury. Finally, too many people buy into the 'no pain, no gain' mindset. On longs runs you may well feel fatigued, or may even get a bit of burning in your thighs or calves, but any actual pain should be taken as a warning sign that something is wrong, and should be acted upon immediately. Overuse injuries don't happen suddenly: there will always be warning pain, and that warning pain should never be ignored. It won't magically disappear if you try to push through it: it'll get worse and seriously curtail your training. End the session immediately, ice the affected area, and seek professional advice.

Burying your head in the sand about an injury and just hoping it'll go away is the worst possible thing to do. After a great winter of training in 2007/2008, I was flying. I set personal best scores in the lab, was as lean as I'd ever been, and was winning races. I felt bombproof. I then went away for a week's training in the mountains outside Seville, and straight from a day sitting on trains and planes did a tough workout. I felt a bit of a niggle on the outside of my right knee, but pushed on through and thought nothing of it. As the week went on the pain got more persistent, but stupidly I carried on training. By the end of the week I couldn't walk without it flaring up, but with one of my focus races for the year, the Three Peaks Fell Race, only a week away, I ignored all of my own advice, ran through the pain and hoped it'd miraculously hold up on race day. Unsurprisingly it didn't, and after having to pull out on the first descent my poor long-suffering wife had to deal with me sulking all the way home. Still in denial, I refused to seek proper help and instead turned to on-line self-diag-nosis and running sessions that usually ended with me hobbling home. Eventually, a combination of my wife and my coach dishing out some very

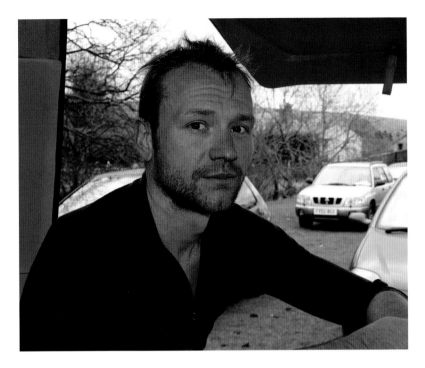

A miserable author after having to pull out of the Three Peaks race

firm tough love persuaded me to see a physio. Within four weeks of seeing him I was back running pain free but, because of my stupidity, I had effectively wasted three times that amount of training.

COMMON RUNNING INJURIES

The following list of six injuries is not comprehensive, but does represent the commonest ailments that tend to befall runners. Self-treatment tips are provided, but, as illustrated by my tale of woe, the fastest route to getting running again is seeking professional advice as soon as you can.

Twisted ankle

You're running along when, with a sickening crunch, you go over on your ankle. Known as a sprain, the ligaments around your ankle are stretched or even torn. Most commonly, you'll go over on the outside of your foot, known as an inversion sprain, but it is possible to also roll your ankle inwards. Once you've hobbled home, immediately put the RICE protocol into action:

R **is for Rest**: Get off your ankle and try not to put any weight on it.

I **is for Ice**: Apply an ice pack, or bag of frozen peas, to your ankle for 15 minutes. Repeat every two hours. Do not apply the pack directly to the skin.

C **is for Compression**: A Tubigrip-style bandage that is tight round the ankle and extends from your toes to just below your knee is ideal.

E **is for Elevation**: Take advantage of gravity to reduce bleeding and swelling. Put your feet up and get someone else to wait on you.

Get to your local Minor Injuries Unit or GP as soon as you're able. They'll be able to access the severity of the sprain and decide whether it merits an X-ray to check for possible fractures.

Once the initial pain and swelling have subsided, take advice from a physio, who'll be able to prescribe a rehab programme. Your ankle will be weak, and the link between your brain and the joint, known as proprioception, compromised. If you don't rehabilitate the ankle properly with wobble-board work and other exercises, you'll be liable to sprain it repeatedly in the future.

Iliotibial Band Syndrome (Runner's knee)

Often known as IT or ITB Syndrome, this overuse injury is characterized by pain on the outside of the knee. The iliotibial band (ITB) is a sheath of thick, fibrous connective tissue that runs down the outside of the thigh and attaches to the hip bone at the top and shinbone at the bottom. If the band is too tight it can flick over a bony prominence on the outside of the knee and become inflamed.

ITB Syndrome typically comes on very slowly, and in its early stages the pain will often not come on until later on during a run. If ignored, though, it will get progressively worse, with persistent pain, even when not running, that is very hard to get rid of.

As soon as the telltale pain on the outside of the knee appears, stop running, return home and ice the affected area. Book in straight away to see a physio, and in the meantime work on your stretching routine and use a foam roller to work on your ITB.

The physio will work on loosening off the ITB with massage techniques that, although painful, are usually effective. He or she should also assess the cause of the problem and prescribe rehab exercises and stretches. In most cases ITB Syndrome is caused by the ITB having to overwork in order to compensate for weak muscles in your buttocks. This weakness is largely caused by sitting, and the strengthening routine, especially the single-legged squats, should protect you from this stubborn and debilitating condition.

Plantar fasciitis

The plantar fascia is a broad, thick band of tissue that runs from under the heel to the front of the foot. The condition is identified by pain under the heel and sometimes along the arch. The pain is often worse first thing in the morning, as the fascia tightens overnight, and will often partially subside as you get going and your foot warms up. As the condition becomes more severe the pain will worsen and won't subside.

Icing and rest are the immediate treatments, but a physio should be consulted at the first signs of this condition. Biomechanical issues and imbalances are usually the cause and should always be addressed with a strengthening and stretching programme before resorting to quick fixes such as orthotics, heavily supportive shoes or even night splints. Again, the strengthening work in the plan and the progressive approach should protect you from this condition.

Patellofemoral Pain Syndrome

This is a generic term to cover a number of ailments that are characterized by pain at the front of the knee. Often flaring up when descending stairs or running downhill, the usual cause is a problem with the tracking of the kneecap, resulting in damage and inflammation of the surrounding and associated tissues. The pain may be an aching in the joint, there may be swelling after activity, and sitting for long periods may be uncomfortable.

Apply the RICE protocol and make an appointment with a physio. There will often be a tightness or an imbalance in the thigh muscles causing the kneecap to track incorrectly. The physio will use massage techniques to release tight tissues, and maybe infrared or heat treatment to reduce inflammation. They will then look for reasons for the imbalances, which often include weak buttock muscles caused by, you've guessed it, sitting. A stretching and strengthening routine that will be very similar to the one in the plan will be prescribed.

Achilles' tendonitis

The Achilles' tendon attaches the large muscles of your calf to your heel bone. Achilles' tendonitis can either be acute or chronic. The acute condition comes on over a matter of a few days, typically following a sudden increase in training volume or intensity. The pain will usually be felt just above the ankle bone, and the area will be tender to the touch. It'll often be present at the onset of exercise, but ease as the session goes on, and will tend to respond well to rest. With the chronic condition, the pain will develop slowly over a matter of weeks or months and will often be more noticeable walking up hills or stairs. There may be nodules or lumps in the tendon, it will be tender to the touch, and there may be swelling or thickening.

For both conditions, adopt the RICE protocol. If the condition is chronic, or is acute but doesn't respond to RICE, make an appointment with a physio. The commonest cause of Achilles' tendonitis is too much, too soon, or a new training stimulus that the body simply isn't used to. This could be extra distance, increased pace, an unusually hilly run, or even running barefoot on sand. Weak and tight calf muscles are often to blame, and the physio will be able to relieve this tightness, prescribe strengthening and stretching exercises, and work on the actual tendon.

Additionally, I know many runners who have suffered from Achilles' tendonitis who swear by long compression socks. They will certainly help to keep the tendon warmer, and there's growing evidence for the merits of compression clothing. If you don't mind the 'Paula Radcliffe look', they're definitely worth a try.

Shin splints

As a general term, shin splints refers to any pain at the front of the lower leg. However, an actual shin splint is characterized by a pain at the front inside of the shin bone. The pain will often be present at the commencement of exercise, ease as the session continues, but then return after the activity and, if ignored, become more severe and persistent. There is sometimes swelling, pain to the touch and lumps and bumps along the inside of the shin.

In the early stages of the condition RICE can be very effective in conjunction with focused stretching of the lower leg. Seeing a physio early on can definitely help speed up recovery and is strongly recommended. There can often be a biomechanical cause to the condition, and a good physio will be able to advise you as to the best rehab exercises to prevent a recurrence. Running excessively on hard pavements is often to blame, and a simple switch to off-road running combined with some physio can provide a quick and effective cure.

As with Achilles' tendonitis, many runners find compression socks or calf guards to be effective in the rehab and prevention of shin splints.

WHO TO SEE

For almost all running niggles and non-traumatic sports injuries, my first port of call would always be an experienced sports physio. The sports distinction is very important. They will be familiar with the condition you're presenting to them, and will realize the importance of getting you running again. They'll also know that, in all but the most extreme cases, simply telling you to rest is not an option. They'll discuss suitable cross-training options, and actively involve you in the treatment and recovery from your injury. There's no reason for you to lose significant amounts of fitness while recovering. A good sports physio should give you the tools to go away and deal with your injury, and not just set you up for a long series of costly treatments. Look for personal recommendations by speaking to local runners and looking at local running club on-line message boards.

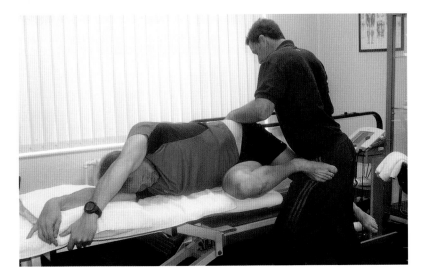

Physio

There is a plethora of other therapists offering their services to injured runners, including osteopaths and chiropractors. Although I've had some great treatments from both of these types of practitioners, they only seem to fix the symptoms without addressing the underlying causes. This means you end up in a constant cycle of treatment, and never escape the therapist's couch. If you know an osteopath or chiropractor whom you trust and who is familiar with your body, they can be invaluable in a must-be-on-that-start-line situation, but I'd always recommend a sports physio first.

MASSAGE

Sports massage should have a regular place in your training plan. I'd personally love to be able to afford one every week but tend to make do with one a month. As well as being incredibly relaxing, it's the equivalent of a regular MOT of my body, and provides valuable information about areas of tightness and potential problems. Regular problem areas can be treated and kept under control, and I'm convinced that regular massage is one of the secrets to injury prevention. Too many runners turn to a massage therapist once they're already injured, but I believe their true value is preventative. First check who the masseur or masseuse is affiliated to. There are basically two governing bodies:, the Institute of Sport and Remedial Massage (ISRM), and the Sports Massage Association (SMA). Ask to see their qualifications, how long their training course was, what the last career development course they attended was, and if they have any references from past clients. Again, your local running club can be a valuable resource for personal recommendations. I'd also tend to look for a masseur or masseuse who was full-time, as they have more hands-on time and usually a greater range of clients.

Although it'll never be as good as the real thing, and you

Massage

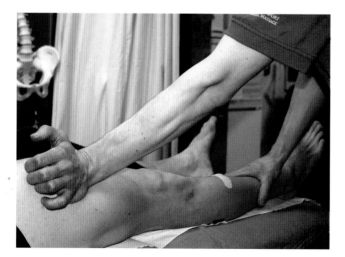

won't get the feedback about the state of your body, self-massage can be an effective way of keeping on top of tight muscles. Products such as foam rollers and the Stick *www.thestick.net* can be used while you're sitting in front of the TV, and certainly won't do you or your running any harm.

Spotting the Signs of Overtraining

You can do too much of a good thing, and with other demands on your life such as work and family sometimes adding to the strain, training can become counter-productive and start weakening your body. The plan is designed to be progressive, and as long as you pay close attention to session duration and intensity, and adhere to rest days, overtraining shouldn't be a problem. However, everyone is different and, with varying physiological make-ups and different levels of non-exercise stresses, keeping an eye out for the classic signs of overtraining is essential. If you find yourself exhibiting more than two or three of the signs described for more than a couple of consecutive days, take an extra rest day and reduce training volume by 50 per cent for the rest of that week. Try to reduce other stresses that may be impacting on your training, and if necessary repeat that training week rather than moving ahead. As well as logging your training, keep a daily note of these factors, and be aware of any sudden changes or lasting trends.

PERSISTENT ILLNESS

Up to a certain level, training has a beneficial effect on your immune system, but push too hard and it can lower your body's defences. Factor in breathing in large volumes of air, especially if you're training in a public gym, and you can significantly increase your risk of upper respiratory tract infections. A few colds and sniffles are almost inevitable if you're training over the winter, but if you find you're not shifting them or are picking up more than usual it might be time to back off. Knowing whether to train or not if you're feeling a bit under the weather can be difficult, but if in doubt, don't. I've always followed the advice that if your symptoms are above neck level then trying light training is okay, but if you have symptoms below the neck, such as a chesty cough, muscular aches or a temperature, training is an absolute no-no.

RESTING HEART RATE

Getting into the habit of checking your pulse first thing in the morning is an excellent way of detecting the early warning signs of overtraining or a looming illness. Once you've got over the shock of your alarm going off, lie back and relax for a minute and find your radial (wrist) pulse. Count the beats in a minute and note them down in your training log. You can just count for 30 or even 15 seconds and multiply by two and four respectively, but a full minute gives a more accurate reading. After a week or so you should get a good idea of what your typical resting heart rate is. As your training progresses, expect to see your resting pulse steadily dropping. However, if you notice an increase or decrease in rate from one day to another of more than five beats per minute, take a rest day or only train very lightly.

RAPID WEIGHT LOSS

For most people, losing a bit of fat should be one of the biggest bonuses of training to run a marathon, but too rapid weight loss is a sign of overtraining and indicates that you're losing muscle tissue as well as fat. Daily weigh-ins and plotting your weight on a graph is the best way to monitor your weight. Make sure you weigh yourself at the same time each day. Expect to see daily fluctuations of up to or even over 1 kg, but if the overall trend shows weight loss of much more than that from one week to the next it's possible you're overtraining. Obviously, some people initially have more fat to lose than others and can expect to see more rapid weight loss, but any sudden significant increase in the rate of weight loss should be viewed with suspicion.

POOR SLEEP

I can guarantee that most of you starting running will sleep better than you've ever slept, but having sleeping problems is a classic sign of overtraining. As sleep is when your body repairs itself and recovers, not sleeping throws you into a vicious circle. Typically, an athlete who's suffering from overtraining has trouble getting to sleep, owing to restless legs or just feeling wide awake. As well as maybe backing off your training for a couple of days, look at your bedtime routine and sleeping environment. If possible, avoid training within two hours of going to bed or, if you have to train late, factor in a relaxing stretching session when you get in, followed by a hot bath. Drink some hot milk, but avoid tea or coffee any later than midday. Avoid watching TV or going on the computer in the bedroom or immediately before going to bed. Make sure your bedroom is quiet, genuinely dark and not too warm. If you are struggling to sleep, don't lie there stressing and watching the clock. Get up, make yourself some warm milk, read for half an hour and then try going back to bed.

EXCESSIVE MUSCLE SORENESS

DOMS (Delayed Onset Muscle Soreness) is characterized by soreness in your muscles 48–72 hours after exercise. It's caused by the microtraumas that occur in your muscle tissue following a new training load. It's perfectly normal, and the process of repairing the muscle damage is how muscles become stronger. You'll probably find you experience a bad case of the DOMS the first couple of times you do the strengthening routine. Over 24 hours the soreness normally fades, and exercise and recovery techniques can speed up this process. If you're consistently overdoing it, though, the soreness will not ease, and your legs will feel continuously sore, heavy and tired. Back off running for a couple of days, and do some non-impact, non-weight bearing exercise such as swimming.

IRRITABILITY AND POOR MOOD

Exercise should improve your mood and give you a genuine mental lift. As well as the very real 'Runner's High', produced by chemicals in your brain released during exercise, sticking to a regular training plan will improve feelings of self-worth and give a genuine sense of achievement. Too much training, combined with not enough recovery and insufficient sleep, can really bring you down, though. As well as feeling irritable, snappy or a bit low, one of the classic signs of overtraining is genuinely starting to dread training sessions. We all have days when getting out to train is a real effort but, in the main, you should look forward to it. This plan provides far more variety of exercise than most running programmes, and if you find you're consistently struggling with motivation then maybe you need to ease off for a couple of days.

The Plan

	Week 9	Week 10	Week 11	Week 12
Monday	Recovery session. Yoga/pilates or rest	Recovery session. Yoga/pilates or rest	Recovery session. Yoga/pilates or rest	Recovery session. Yoga/pilates or rest
Tuesday	Run 1: 20 mins tempo (10–**5**–5) Followed by strength routine	Run 1: 22 mins tempo (10–**7**–5) Followed by strength routine	Run 1: 25 mins tempo (10–**10**–5) Followed by strength routine	Run 1: 27 mins tempo (10–**12**–5) Followed by strength routine
Wednesday	30 mins swim	30 mins swim	30 mins swim	30 mins swim
Thursday	Run 2: Intervals 2 x 3 mins (3 mins reco) Followed by strength routine	Run 2: Intervals 2 x 4 mins (3 mins reco) Followed by strength routine	Run 2: Intervals 3 x 4 mins (3 mins reco) Followed by strength routine	Run 2: Intervals 2 x 5 mins (3 mins reco) Followed by strength routine
Friday	Rest day	Rest day	Rest day	Rest day
Saturday	Run 3: LSD 40 mins	Run 3: LSD 45 mins	Run 3: LSD 50 mins	Run 3: 20 mins jog in race kit
Sunday	Cycle 60 mins	Cycle 60 mins	Cycle 60 mins	10 km race/run

The Sessions

MONDAY

This remains a rest day or a recovery session. After two long sessions at the weekend, it'd be an ideal day to book in for a massage. If you're feeling at all tired or heavy legged, take a complete day off or go for a gentle wallow in the pool.

TUESDAY

Tuesday is a tempo session followed by the strength routine. Throughout Level 1 you've been working on finding your 6/10 comfortable running pace. Tempo running is all about getting you used to 'sustainable discomfort' and discovering that you have additional gears on top of your steady running pace. By starting to work at a faster pace regularly, your comfortable pace will start to feel even easier and start to become faster. The pace should only be fractionally higher than your comfortable pace and score 7–7.5/10. You should still be able to talk, but only in short sentences, and you should be having to concentrate to maintain the effort. The first figure in the brackets refers to your easy-paced warm-up in minutes, the second bold figure is the 'tempo time', and the final figure is your cool down.

WEDNESDAY

Swimming will be an ideal recovery after your tempo run.

THURSDAY

This is an interval session followed by the strength routine. You've already done some interval training at the start of Level 1, with the walk and run workouts, but now we're using them to increase running intensity. As with the tempo workout, the idea is to use faster paced running to develop your steady-state running. Your pace should be fractionally higher than the tempo session, pushing your effort level to 8–8.5/10. You'll probably be able to manage single-word answers, but not much more. Pace the intervals so that your running speed remains consistent through the whole workout. Don't hammer the first minute of the first interval. If anything, start off at about tempo pace and build gradually through the interval. Start off the session with five minutes of brisk walking followed by five minutes of easy-paced running. You'll be doing two three-minute intervals with three minutes of walking recovery between them: 2 X 3 mins (3 mins reco). Finish off with three minutes of walking followed by seven minutes of easy jogging to cool down, before going into the strength routine.

FRIDAY
This is a compulsory and much deserved rest day.

SATURDAY
This is your LSD run. This is where you go back to your 6/10 effort level and build your running stamina and endurance. Remember to start getting used to hydrating on the go, and if you get the chance get off the roads and onto the trails.

SUNDAY
This is cycling day. You've got a rest day or recovery workout on Monday, so if you've got the energy feel free to ride fairly hard or take a spinning class. If Saturday's run took it out of you, though, use low gears, choose a flat course, and go for an easy spin. A complete rest day isn't an option, though, as a ride will do your legs some good.

CHAPTER 3

Level 3: Weeks 13–20

Introduction

Breaking through 10 km, or about an hour of continuous running, is a massive achievement that you should be really proud of. You should be really starting to feel like a runner now. The tempo and interval sessions will have given you extra running gears, your easy-paced speed will have increased, and you should be able to take a variety of terrains in your stride. You're now ready to take on the challenge of a half marathon.

Don't be intimidated by the 'M' word; you've got eight weeks to build on the rock solid running foundations you've already laid, and by the time you've completed this block of training you'll be more than prepared for 13.1 miles of running. The basic structure of your training week remains consistent, with the main emphasis being on you simply building the ability to run for longer. We introduce using a heart rate monitor for more accurate pacing of workouts, and with runs getting longer cover key areas such as nutrition, recovery and tapering. We also go into some of the not so pleasant and potentially painful aspects of running, and give you tried and tested solutions to avoid them. Finally, with many UK based runners training for the London Marathon and other spring races, much of this and the next block will be through the worst of the British winter. We discuss how you can beat the elements, ensure your safety and keep your training moving forwards.

Heart Rate Training

For the first two blocks of the plan you've been relying on how you felt, your ability to talk, and an exertion score based on these factors to judge your running pace. This will have given you an excellent feel for your own body and a valuable awareness of how your body reacts to running and changes of running intensity. Now you have that understanding, though, I'd strongly recommend that you start using a heart rate monitor.

A heart rate monitor consists of an unobtrusive chest transmitter strap that is worn directly next to the skin and a watch-style monitor that conveniently shows you the important heart rate information. I like to think of heart rate monitors as being a bit like a rev counter on a car. They're an objective way of knowing if you're pushing too hard on a long run, or taking it too easy on a tempo run or interval workout. I don't like novice runners to use a heart rate monitor from day one, as I believe that learning to feel and assess your own pace is a vital running skill. Without a decent base of running fitness, even a short amount of running can make the heart rate go disproportionately high, which can prove very discouraging. Finally, to find accurate heart rate training zones, you need to be able to run continuously for at least 15 minutes. With 12 weeks of solid running training behind you, all of those boxes are ticked, and now is the ideal time to start training with a heart rate monitor.

Buying a heart rate monitor can be a bewildering experience. Knowing which features are relevant to your training needs and how much to spend is a potential minefield. It's all too easy to end up with a monitor with an instruction manual that needs weeks to get through and a degree in electrical engineering to understand. In the majority of cases, features such as fitness tests and automatic zone setting are largely superfluous and often wildly inaccurate. You're far better off focusing on key, but less glamorous features, such as being able to manually set training zones, and decent session recall, including time spent in the desired training zone. There are now many manufacturers producing heart rate monitors, and it's possible to get a budget monitor for well under £30. However, for reliability of performance and post-sale service, I'd strongly recommend sticking to well-known brands such as Polar, Suunto and, if you also want GPS distance/speed logging, Garmin.

Without GPS, £70–£100 will get you a monitor from one of the top brands with all the features you need.

The classic method for calculating heart rate training zones is to use a formula such as 220-age to estimate maximal heart rate and then work out percentage bands from that figure. There are other formulae that claim to be more accurate by factoring in resting heart rate, but they're all very crude approximations and, because sedentary subjects were often used to derive them, they usually deliver significantly lower maximal heart rate values than reality, and therefore all training zones calculated from them are skewed low. It's important to note that automatic zone calculator functions on heart rate monitors also use variations of the 220-age formula, and shouldn't be applied.

Some people advocate field testing of maximal heart rate to get an accurate figure. Simply put, this normally involves finding a hill and running up it as hard as you can until you feel as though you're going to explode or pass out. As well as being extremely unpleasant, and potentially dangerous without medical supervision, it's often far from accurate. Very few people are able to push themselves to their absolute maximum, and it only takes a fractional drop in your psychological or physiological condition to significantly skew your result.

The ideal method for establishing accurate heart rate training zones is to book in for a testing session at a sports science laboratory. Although you may feel that this is the preserve of elite athletes, professional sports testing has become much more accessible and more affordable for amateur athletes. I'd always argue that amateur athletes almost have more to gain from one of these sessions than full-time pros. You're devoting a lot of time and effort to your training, as well as balancing it with work and family commitments, and you deserve to do everything you can to maximize the effectiveness of your precious training hours. A typical lab-based running test and analysis will take approximately two hours and will generally cost around £100. Protocols vary slightly, but you will generally be expected to run on a treadmill for around 20–30 minutes. This will include a warm-up, a sub-maximal test, and finally a push to your maximum. Throughout the test the composition of your exhaled air will be analysed, and this allows the sports scientist to accurately assess your body's response to exercise. During the sub-maximal part of the testing you'll find crucial information about your running economy and your body's ability to burn fat as a fuel. This part of the test will also show you your heart rate at threshold, and it's from this key bit of information that your heart rate zones are calculated. Threshold is the intensity at which your body is going into the red, and from a distance running perspective is vital. In comparison, the maximal part of the test, which gives a figure known as VO2, is far less important. VO2 refers to your body's ability to uptake and use oxygen, and although it's the stat that endurance athletes will always ask about, threshold is far more important. It therefore doesn't really matter if you're unable or unwilling to push yourself to absolute failure. There are labs offering testing throughout the country, and you should be looking for one that is BASES (British Association of Sport and Exercise Science) accredited. Go to *www.bases.org.uk/labfinder.asp* to find one near you.

If the idea of a lab test seems a bit over the top to you, there's an easy-to-perform field test that can be used to determine your heart rate at threshold, and from that you can calculate personal and accurate heart rate training zones.

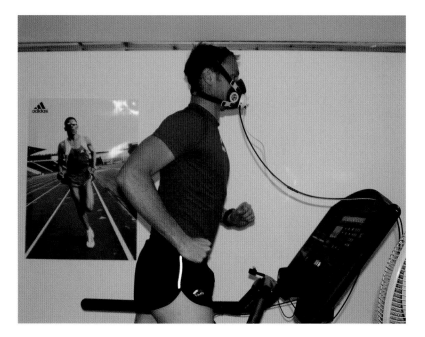

The author in the lab

You'll need a flat running route without any obstructions (a running track is best), and a heart rate monitor that allows you to recall average heart rate.

Have a complete rest day the day before the test, don't eat for two hours beforehand, and make sure you're well hydrated. This test can be conducted as your tempo session in Week 13 of the plan.

✓ Warm-up for 10 minutes, building up your heart rate progressively.
✓ Complete 6 X 50 m acceleration strides with 30 seconds recovery. These are not all-out sprints, just purposeful strides at 60–70 per cent of sprinting pace.
✓ Start the recorder of your heart rate monitor and run as hard as you sustainably can for 15 minutes. Don't go off too hard, and try to pace your effort so you cover as far as you can manage in the time. Stop the recorder on your heart rate monitor at the end of the 15 minutes.
✓ Cool down with 10 minutes of easy jogging.
✓ Your average heart rate for the 15 minutes will equate to your threshold. Note down that figure.

Apply these percentage bands to your threshold heart rate figure:

Zone 1: 60–85%
Zone 2: 85–89%
Zone 3: 90–94%
Zone 4: 95–99%

Once you've got your training zones, you need to know how to apply them to training sessions.

TEMPO SESSIONS
Warm-up: Zone 1 building to Zone 2 during the second 5 minutes.
Tempo block: Zone 3.
Cool down: Zone 1 easing right back to a walk and sub-Zone 1 for final 1–2 minutes.

INTERVAL SESSIONS

Warm-up: Zone 1 building to Zone 2 during the second 5 minutes.

Work interval: Upper Zone 3 pushing well into Zone 4 by the end of the interval.

Rest interval: Returning to Zones 1–2.

Cool down: Zone 1 easing right back to a walk and sub-Zone 1 for final 1–2 minutes.

LSD RUNS

The whole run should be in Zones 1–2, allowing the heart rate to rise to mid to upper Zone 2 on uphills, but not pushing into Zone 3. This is the session that will require the most discipline, but as staying in these zones develops your running economy and endurance it's vital not to let your heart rate creep into Zone 3. You might feel as though it's better to run harder and that you will get fitter by doing so, but all you'll be doing is exposing yourself to unnecessary injury risk and not addressing the most crucial area of fitness for a successful marathon.

During training sessions it's essential to stay strictly within the designated zone. It's quite possible that you'll feel as though you're working harder, or more likely easier, in the sessions using heart rate than when you were using perceived effort. Don't worry about this, it's perfectly normal and you'll quickly adapt and get used to them. Many heart rate monitors allow you to set an audible alarm to let you know if you're above or below your target zone, and this can be a really useful function. Many people make the mistake of relying on average heart rate recall, and having done a session without barely a glance at the monitor think that, because their average heart rate was within their target zone, they've ticked the box for that session. However, it's perfectly possible to get an average heart rate figure bang in the middle of your target zone without having actually spent any time in the zone. A good analogy is a man with one foot in a bucket of iced water and the other foot in a bucket of boiling water. He's not averagely comfortable, is he? The crucial post-workout heart rate information is time spent in the target zone, and to maximize that you need to be constantly aware of, and checking, your heart rate.

Fuelling your Training

GENERAL NUTRITION

Although many people start running with the aim of losing weight, you definitely don't want to be attempting to train for a marathon in conjunction with any form of restrictive dieting. You wouldn't try to run your car without petrol, would you? Equally, training for a marathon does not give you free rein to eat and drink what you want with complete abandon. An 80 kg man running at 10-minute mile pace for an hour will burn about 800 kcals, but feeling smug and virtuous back at the office after his run he gobbles down a King Size Mars Bar and instantly wipes out over half of those burnt calories. As dull as it sounds, a sensible, varied diet including plenty of lean meat, fruit, vegetables, and unrefined (brown and wholegrain) carbohydrates is the best way to fuel your training. It's also important to keep well hydrated. Cut back on junk calories from foods and drinks high in refined sugars or unsaturated fats, and snack healthily on fruit, nuts and seeds. Don't limit your food intake, but equally don't use your running as an excuse to binge. If you're a vegetarian or vegan, make sure you are taking in an adequate amount of complete proteins, or your body won't be able to recover fully from workouts, but a balanced meat-free diet can definitely fuel marathon training. I'm a big believer in keeping a food diary, as I find that having to write down everything I eat tends to make me stop and think before putting something in my mouth. For example, as I'm writing this I'm currently training 10–15 hours per week in preparation for the World Duathlon Championships, and yesterday, which is a typical weekday, I trained/ate/drank as follows:

0700
✓ Espresso and 250 ml of water

0730–0830
✓ 60 mins morning run

0840 Breakfast
✓ 500 ml water

- ✓ Espresso
- ✓ Wholegrain bagel with butter
- ✓ Poached egg

1100
- ✓ 500 ml water
- ✓ Cup of tea
- ✓ Apple

1300 Lunch
- ✓ 500 ml water
- ✓ Cup of tea
- ✓ Tuna, salad and mayonnaise sandwich made with wholegrain bread
- ✓ Banana

1600
- ✓ 250 ml water
- ✓ Wholegrain bagel with cottage cheese

1800–2000
- ✓ 2-hour bike session
- ✓ 750 ml water
- ✓ 2 energy gels

2015 Dinner
- ✓ 500 ml water
- ✓ Rib eye steak
- ✓ Roasted vegetables (butternut squash, sweet potato and courgette)
- ✓ Apple

I'm 190 cm tall and weigh in around the 80 kg mark, so am not a small guy, but this isn't a vast amount of food. Although a nutritionist could probably find a few flaws (I'll put my hand up to a 'healthy' caffeine addiction), what I'm trying to illustrate is that you don't need to try anything outlandish with your general nutrition, or guzzle vast amounts of pasta.

PRE-TRAINING NUTRITION

Eating before a training session is all about making sure that you've got the right amount of fuel on board and that you've eaten far enough in advance and consumed the right sort of food so it won't affect your training negatively. First of all, lets bust the myth of the 'pasta party'. You don't need to load up on pasta or anything else the day before a long training session, and the same applies to the day before a race. Your body's energy stores can only take a finite amount: anything more will just be stored as fat. Eating a normal sized meal that contains a decent amount of carbohydrates will do the job of topping up those stores. You don't have to slog through a mountain of pasta.

Trying to eat two hours before training is the ideal, and it's a good idea to avoid anything too rich, high in fat, or hard-to-digest protein such as meat or fish. As you can see from my day's food, my pre-training snack is a wholegrain bagel with cottage cheese.

Obviously, if you're training first thing in the morning this can be tough. As you can see from my food diary, my morning run is done in a fasted state. This is fine for sessions of up to 60 minutes and of low intensities (heart rate zones 1–2), and has been shown to improve fat-burning ability. However, as your blood sugar is very low when you wake up, any quality work such as tempo runs/intervals or sessions longer than an hour shouldn't be attempted in a fasted state. In this case a banana, energy gel or energy bar just before heading out can be the solution, and should keep you going for an hour or so. Some people just can't stomach eating anything just before training, though. Experiment with different foods, but if you can't find one that works you may have to consider not training in the morning.

EATING ON THE RUN

For shorter sessions, such as your interval and tempo workout, you shouldn't have to take on any food while running. However, during your LSD run you'll need to top up your fuel reserves. Your mantra should be 'early, little and often'. During a long session it's vital to start taking fuel on almost right from the off rather than leaving it until you feel as though you need it. Like waiting until you're thirsty before taking water on board, if you wait until you're hungry it'll be too late and meeting the Wall, or as cyclists call it, 'bonking', is inevitable.

On long runs and rides I'll be eating from as soon as 30 minutes into the

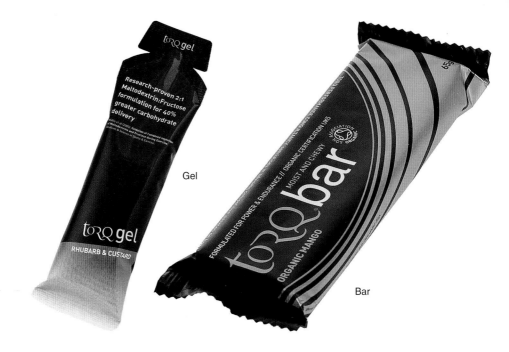

Gel

Bar

session. The accepted wisdom for how much you need to eat is 1 g of carbo-hydrate per kg of bodyweight per hour. For me at 80 kg, this usually translates into one 37 g gel giving 28 g of carbs on the half hour, and a 65 g energy bar on the hour delivering 42 g of carbs. This brings me in 10 g short, but I'll often mix in some carb-based sports drink with my water. As well as helping keep my electrolyte salts topped up, this gives me the rest of the energy I need.

If you do decide to use a sports drink, it's important to make sure it isn't too concentrated, as this will inhibit absorption and potentially contribute to dehydrating you. Six per cent is generally considered to be the optimum concentration, and most powdered brands give instructions on how to mix to these levels. Beware of some pre-mixed brands, though, as they often come in much higher concentrations.

What and how much you can tolerate when running is a very individual thing. Your LSD runs are when you should be experimenting with brands and flavours of gels, bars and sports drinks, timing taking on your nutrition, amounts and how to balance it with your fluid intake. By the time you get to the end of this half marathon block, your fuelling strategy should be set in stone and totally effective. If you're not getting on with sports-specific bars or gels, try breakfast cereal bars, malt loaf or even drip-feeding yourself jelly babies. I know one runner who's incredibly successful over marathons and ultras who swears by a quarter of a sandwich every 30 minutes made with honey and cheap white bread with the crusts cut off. Along with consistency in training and avoiding injury, getting your marathon day fuelling right is of paramount importance to your success over 26.2 miles.

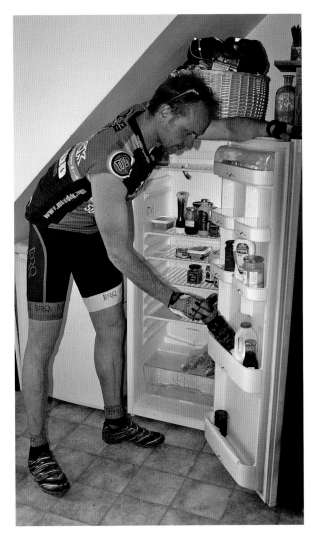

Have your post long ride or run recovery drink made-up ready

POST-RUN NUTRITION

You'll notice from my food diary that, within 15–20 minutes of my sessions finishing, I'm eating a meal containing both carbohydrates and protein. This is vital to kick-start your body's recovery process, and there's a golden 20-minute window immediately post-exercise when your body is crying out for nutrition. Any carbs will be sucked up and used to replenish your body's depleted stores, and protein will immediately be sent into action helping muscles grow, repair and recover.

Unfortunately, a meal isn't always practical immediately after training, and especially following a long session when you've probably been hitting bars and gels, not always easy to stomach. This is often the case for me after my long weekend rides and runs, and to solve the problem I'll have a recovery shake made up and waiting in the fridge for me. There are a number available either in powder form or pre-mixed, and finding a brand and flavour that suits you is down to experimentation. What they all have in common is a blend of protein and easily available carbohydrates designed to optimize your post-workout recovery. A full-portion recovery drink is probably overkill after sessions of up to an hour but, for longer workouts, it's essential. Commercial recovery drinks can be expensive, but there's a cheap and simple solution: 500 ml of semi-skimmed milk blended with a banana provides exactly what your body needs at a fraction of the price. For shorter sessions, if you're not able to eat straight away, take a half portion of recovery drink, or 250 ml of semi-skimmed milk with half a banana.

Runners who are trying to lose weight often worry about the extra calories that post-run nutrition involves. However, if you leave your body hungry, you'll be ravenously hungry three to four hours after your session, and almost guaranteed to eat far more on top of your normal food than the extra calories contained in a recovery drink. This is often the reason for the surprisingly common phenomenon of people gaining weight when training for a marathon. They'll go for their long Sunday run, not have a recovery drink for fear of the additional calories, but then go on a mad and often uncontrollable feeding frenzy later in the day. This was happening to a friend of mine who, despite training hard, was still gaining weight and had a seemingly insatiable appetite. Half a banana and a glass of milk post-training solved his problem and, within a week, he was starting to finally shift some weight. As well as making weight gain more likely, if you ignore post-run nutrition you'll be seriously compromising your recovery, which will have a knock-on effect on future training sessions, and therefore on your fitness gains.

SUPPLEMENTATION

There are plenty of supplements available that claim to boost running performance, help you lose weight while you train, or stop you getting colds and sniffles. I've always been deeply sceptical of such claims, and apart from a multivitamin and mineral to cover my bases don't see the need to pop numerous pills and potions. Stick to the training plan, eat sensibly, and you'll become a better runner, probably lose some weight and, without spending money on pills, save yourself a lot of money. If you're struggling with the programme, or find you're getting ill more than normal, seek professional medical advice rather than self-medicating.

ALCOHOL

You don't need to be teetotal to be a marathon runner, and moderate alcohol consumption doesn't necessarily adversely affect your training or performance. Members of the worldwide Hash House Harriers Running Clubs are known as 'drinkers with a running problem'. There are a couple of factors to be aware of, though, before ordering that pint or pouring that glass of wine. The first is that alcohol contains a lot of empty calories that the body will tend to store as fat. One of the most effective steps many people can take to lose weight is to reduce alcohol consumption. Second, and I've certainly noticed this as I've got older, you can feel even a couple of drinks the morning after, and if getting out from under your duvet for a two-hour run in the freezing rain is a struggle at the best of times, a sore head isn't going to help. I tend to find that when I'm training hard, my desire to drink becomes less, and the thought of the training session I've got planned the next morning, always strengthens my resolve. That said, a summer's evening run or ride will often finish at my local for a rehydrating pint – apparently the electrolyte balance is perfect – and I've been known to have a pint of beer or glass of wine the night before a big race to ease my nerves. Making something a forbidden fruit only makes it more tempting, so my advice is not to try to inflict a blanket ban on yourself, but just to be sensible.

Recovery

I touched on the importance of optimizing your recovery when discussing post-run nutrition, but as well as getting your recovery drink straight down your throat there are a number of other techniques you can use to help your legs recover after a long run. As well as providing your body with the fuel it needs to replenish and repair itself, you're looking to address any tightnesses or imbalances that may have built up, aid blood flow back to the heart to remove waste metabolites from your muscles and prevent blood pooling, and to help reduce the infamous DOMS.

You feel okay after a gruelling race or training session; a bit tired, but your legs don't feel too bad. The next day, though, or even the day after that, your muscles are stiff and sore, and you're hobbling around like an octogenarian. Welcome to the painful world of DOMS.

DOMS tends to flare up 24–48 hours after unusually tough or unaccustomed exercise. It'll usually ease after 72 hours. Although the exact mechanisms still aren't fully understood, microtrauma to the actual muscle fibres is the most likely cause. The old theory of it being caused by lactic acid has been disproved. Novel exercise stimuli, like the first time you worked through the strengthening routine, probably elicit the strongest effect, but with repeat exposure the effects dramatically and rapidly diminish.

Reduce DOMS by introducing new training methods, or by upping intensity gradually, as we do in this programme, and adopting a good recovery routine, but if you are suffering from a bout reassure yourself that the healing mechanism is what makes your muscles become stronger.

STRETCHING

Post-exercise stretching for injury prevention and performance gains is still a matter of hot debate. However, in a recovery context, the positive evidence is much stronger. Working on typically tight areas such as hip flexors and glutes can make all the difference as to how you feel the day after a long run. As we discussed in Level 1, the best time to work through your stretching routine is immediately after your run finishes, but this isn't always practical. If you've just finished a long run in the worst of winter weather, rolling around on the floor for 10–20 minutes trying to stretch is the last thing you're going to want to do. Have your recovery drink, have a hot bath or shower, get some comfy clothing on, and then have a bit of a stretch. If even that feels too much, another really effective recovery technique is just to lie down with your feet up against a wall for 10 minutes. This will help pooled blood drain from your legs, and will gently stretch your calves, hamstrings and glutes.

ACTIVE RECOVERY

Although it may seem counter-intuitive that more exercise can help you to recover, going out for a bike ride the day after a long run can do wonders for sore legs. It's no coincidence that Tour de France riders will head out for a two-hour spin on 'rest days'. Exercise increases blood flow and aids the flushing out of metabolic by-products. The benefits of the 'recovery runs' that are often prescribed in more running-centric programmes are more questionable, as even plodding along in zone 1 still involves considerable impact and stressful loading of your muscles. Far better to get on your bike, find a flat course, stick it in the smaller chain-ring and spin your legs out. Your legs might feel a bit stiff and achy for the first five to 10 minutes but I guarantee, by the end of the ride, they'll feel better.

COMPRESSION TIGHTS

First arising in a clinical setting to improve post-operative blood flow, and then being applied to long-haul flights to prevent deep vein thrombosis, compression garments are now common among athletes. In terms of independent research, although several studies have shown equality compared with other recovery techniques, the jury is still out. There's no doubt, though, that the anecdotal evidence is strong, and many top athletes swear by their efficacy. Putting a pair of compression tights on to hang out post-training is certainly no hardship, and your legs can feel noticeably fresher after a good night's kip in them. Personally I'm a big believer in their effectiveness, and donning a pair of compression tights is a key part of my recovery routine. I've found them to be particularly effective when I've had a long drive after a race, or for a lazy Sunday afternoon after a long morning run. You can easily wear them under your normal clothes so, for me, they're a no-brainer. It's important, though, that they are tight enough to give a genuine compressive effect, so buy a quality brand such as Skins or CompresSport, and take care with sizing.

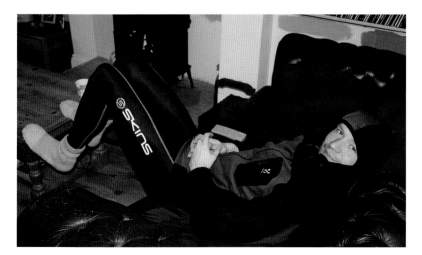

The author recovering in compression tights after long winter run

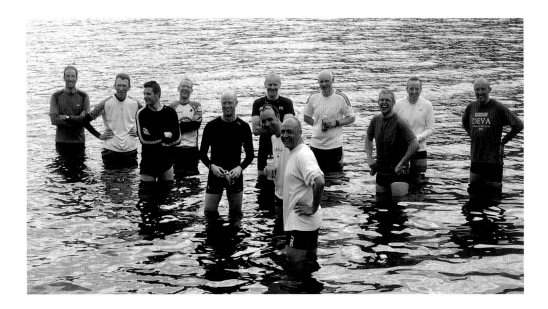

Making the most of
a cold lake on an
Ironman Training
Camp

ICE BATHS

Deeply unpleasant, ice baths have been adopted by elite sportsmen world-wide with surprisingly little research backing. That said, a 2008 study in the International Journal of Sports Medicine showed positive results for cyclists competing in a multi-day stage race who had nightly 14-minute dunkings in 15 °C water. Cold water closes blood capillaries and stops bleeding in damaged muscles. Water pressure can also act like compression tights. (Even a few feet of water adds pressure: dive to the deep end in the pool and feel your goggles squashing your eyeballs.) In addition, cold acts as an analgesic by numbing nerve endings. Sitting in a cold stream after a tough, hot run definitely feels good and won't do you any harm. On the other hand, you're a tougher runner than me if you're willing to sit in a cold bath after a long winter run. If the idea does appeal to you, though, the good news is that the research suggests that tepid water (15–25 °C) is as, if not more, effective than ice cold (<5 °C,) and you only need to do 10–20 minutes.

MASSAGE

This is another universally accepted recovery method. Correct massage technique can increase blood flow, correctly align muscle fibres and scar tissue, and reduce tightness. It's imperative that the therapist understands what training or racing you've been doing, or have coming up, as too deep or aggressive massage can increase muscle damage or reduce performance. I always tend to steer clear of post-race massage tents. You need to think about the benefits immediately after exercise. If you have just completed a very hard race or session and your legs are damaged (you will only feel the full extent 24–48 hours later, owing to DOMS), do you really want someone pressing hard and sticking their fingers into the potentially torn and bleeding muscles? Perhaps five minutes in the nearest river and a massage 48 hours later would be a better plan in those circumstances. I try to have a sports massage every two to four weeks, and see it almost as a regular MOT for my body. My therapist is familiar with my body and can give me a valuable warning of any unusual areas of tightness or imbalances. Self-massage can also help with recovery, and as you'll be working on your own muscles it's almost impossible to go too deep and do any damage. Always try to work with strokes back up your legs and towards your heart. Many runners swear by various tools and gadgets to aid self-massage, and if you find something that feels good and works for you, go for it. A golf ball under your feet can feel blissfully good, sitting and rolling on a tennis ball can do wonders for tight glutes, and a physio's foam roller is a staple for runners who suffer from tight ITBs.

DRUGS

Popping a few painkillers during or after a hard run to prevent next day soreness may seem like a good idea, but you could be doing more harm than good. Studies at Ironman Brazil and the Western States 100 Mile Trail Race showed no benefits to guzzling ibuprofen with regards to perceived discomfort during or after the events. More worryingly, the Western States study showed signs of kidney impairment and endotoxemia (bacteria leaking from the colon into the bloodstream), and also higher levels of tissue inflammation. Painkillers should only be taken under doctor's orders for a specific injury. Research has also shown that the risk of hyponatremia (the potentially fatal dilution of body salts) in endurance athletes increases significantly when taking painkillers, so it's not worth the risk.

Tapering

WHAT IS TAPERING?

You'll notice from looking at the plan that in Week 20, your final week before your half marathon, your training volume and intensity decreases. This is known as a taper, and is designed to deliver you to the start line fresh, strong and raring to go. All top runners will taper towards a major race, and their entire year's training will consist of cycles of building up their training and then backing off before competitions. How much they back off, and for how long, depends on the length of the race they'll be attempting – the longer the race, the longer the taper – and where it sits in their priorities. If it's not a major race, the taper won't be too long so that their training isn't disrupted, and a very minor race might not even get a taper and just be seen as a training session. While you're building up your training, despite all your recovery efforts and rest days, your body will be becoming progressively more taxed and tired. This effect wouldn't have been significant during the first two levels, when workouts were relatively short, but in this block, where you'll be running well past the hour and towards two hours, a short taper is necessary. I want you to put in the best performance you possibly can over 13.1 miles so that we can start to get an idea of your potential over the full marathon, and if your legs are heavy and tired that won't happen.

Tapering gives your body the chance to completely replenish its energy supplies and for its muscles to fully rest, repair and recover from the training you've done. Tapering can almost be seen as a middle ground between resting completely and continuing with full training. Although complete rest would achieve the objectives of letting your body restock and recover, it would leave you feeling lifeless and sluggish come race day. By this stage in the programme your body is used to and expects regular exertion, and suddenly withdrawing this stimulus would be a real shock to it. Even after just a week of complete rest, the effort of trying to spur your legs into action wouldn't be conducive to a decent performance. For longer events such as ultras, an athlete may taper for up to a month, and completely stopping training for this long isn't realistic, and would result in lost fitness. As we've already said, though, full training is also a no-no, as you'd be too fatigued to run well. With this in mind, the approach to take is to reduce training volume over a time period suitable for the target race. For a full marathon this would be two weeks, and as in this case, for a half marathon, one week.

For a short week's taper to a half marathon you'll probably be extremely grateful of the shorter workouts, enjoy them, and feel physically and psychologically refreshed. The short 20-minute jog on the Saturday will give your legs a reminder of what you expect them to do on the Sunday, and give you a chance to double-check your kit. During a longer two-week taper, typical before a full marathon, it's not uncommon to start to worry about losing fitness, begin to feel a bit edgy and irritable, and even to suffer from heavy and tired legs. I've been through month-long tapers before ultras, and my wife will vouch that I become a doubt-ridden and grizzly nightmare. All of this is perfectly normal, and most of the 'symptoms' are psychosomatic and a result of increased pre-race nerves and anxiety. There will also be some psychological and physiological withdrawal from the training you've been doing. It's vital to keep reminding yourself that you're tapering for a reason, and that it'll benefit your race day performance. Most of the little niggles you're feeling, and the dead and tired legs you've got, are in your head, and come race day will vanish. You're not training to gain fitness during your taper, and even if you wanted to top up your fitness you're not going to make any progress at this late stage. Panicked last-minute training might do your mindset some good, but you won't be doing your body, or chances of a decent race, any favours, and you won't improve your fitness. If you've put in the consistent weeks of training that the programme prescribes, you will have laid a perfect foundation for a great race, and tapering is the cherry on the cake. Have faith in the work you've done, ignore the niggling doubts, and enjoy the relative rest. You've earned it.

Blood, Sweat and Fears

There are some less savoury aspects of running that can rear their heads, especially as your runs start getting longer. Although many runners and even more non-runners have horror stories about the physical damage, discomfort and humiliations that running can inflict, most are just myths and hearsay, and with some knowledge, planning and preparation are all totally avoidable.

BLISTERS

Blisters aren't a running inevitability, and having your marathon scuppered by them is totally unnecessary. A blister is simply a burn caused by the heat derived from friction. The friction is typically caused by the rubbing of your shoes or socks against the skin on your feet. The most obvious step in preventing blisters is to make sure there is no rubbing. Shoes should fit correctly, and socks should provide a wicking, soft interface between your feet and your shoes. As I mentioned in Level 1, experiment with a number of brands of quality running socks, and once you find one that suits you buy a load of pairs and be absolutely ruthless about replacing them once they've worn out. Modern running shoes don't require a 'breaking in' period, but if you're trying a new make or model don't head out for an epic run in them straight out of the box. Similarly, even if you're used to a make and model of shoe, don't save a new pair for marathon day. You'd be amazed at how many people do this, and even a fractionally differently aligned row of stitches can be enough to cause a blister.

As a runner, your feet, your contact points with the ground, are the most valuable part of your body. The old-school method of preparing your feet for running was to harden them by rubbing on surgical spirit, and although some runners still swear by this, a more pampering approach is far more effective. Keeping the skin on your feet healthy, soft and flexible makes it far less prone to blistering. Get into the habit of taking extra care to dry your feet, especially between the toes, after baths and showers. Keep an eye out for the telltale signs of fungal infections, such as itchy skin and discolouration or thickening of the nails. Seek medical advice on how to treat any infections at the first sign, as they weaken the skin and make you more prone to sores and blisters. Keep your toenails neatly trimmed, and be watchful of any that show signs of ingrowing. Again, early treatment can prevent an unnecessary lay-off from running. Use a pumice stone to remove any hardened skin, then massage in a moisturizing foot cream. I'll also apply a fairly thick foot cream prior to running to act almost as a lubricant, and to help prevent heat build-up at any rubbing points.

Once running, you'll always get a warning that you're getting a blister. You'll feel a 'hot spot' developing, and that's when you should act. No matter how good you're feeling, how strongly you're running, or even if you're on for a training PB, stop. Take off your shoes and check that your socks aren't bunched up, or if there's an object such as a small stone in your shoe. Have a look where the hot spot is on your foot, and check the corresponding point in your shoe. It's quite possible that the inner lining might have worn away and be causing the rubbing. Have a couple of blister plasters such as Compeed in your bum bag, pack or pocket, and slap one on to get you home. Once home, take time to clean and treat the hot spot and to fully investigate, determine and remedy its cause. If you're unable to find an obvious cause, consider applying a blister plaster to the area as a preventative. Never give a hot spot the chance to become a blister.

If you do succumb to a full-blown blister don't try to burst it if it hasn't already burst. If it has burst, do not try to remove the excess dead skin. Bursting blisters or cutting away skin are recipes for causing infection. Clean and dry the area thoroughly and then apply a blister dressing. These dressings act like a second skin and are designed to be left in place until the blister has healed. They're a real blessing to runners and allow, in all but the most severe cases of blistering, for you to continue running.

BLEEDING NIPPLES AND CHAFING

Like blisters, there's no need for any runner to suffer from either of these conditions. The biggest cause of bleeding nipples is the cheap cotton T-shirts that charity runners have inflicted on them. Cotton will hold water and sweat rather than wicking it away, making the T-shirt cling, rub and take on the qualities of a cheese grater. 'Cotton kills' is an often-heard expression in mountain sports circles because of cotton's water-holding and lack of insulating properties. Running in a cotton T-shirt won't kill you, but it can be extremely painful. On certain days, though – and some people are more prone – even the best quality, technical wicking running T-shirt can still result in painfully rubbed nipples. I tend now, for runs longer than 90 minutes, to put a dab of Vaseline (petroleum jelly) on each nipple, and a plaster over the top: simple, effective and a very sensible precaution.

The worse case of chafing I ever saw was on a 50-mile, overnight, off-road ultra. A friend of mine who was a novice to such events wore a pair of cotton underpants beneath his running tights, despite my warnings. To his credit he hobbled home walking like John Wayne, but only after having to have his underpants cut away and copious amounts of Vaseline applied at the 30-mile checkpoint. Like all chafing, this was completely preventable by wearing properly fitting and designed technical wicking fabrics that draw moisture away from the skin. Chafing is typically caused by skin rubbing on skin, or clothing rubbing on skin, and is exacerbated by moisture. Closely fitting running clothing, especially tights and cycling-style shorts, minimize the scope for rubbing, and moisture-wicking fabrics keep your skin dry. A light covering of a specially designed lubricant such as Body Glide can also help in areas you know are prone to chafing. As with eating and drinking, your long training runs are the time to experiment with what clothing works for you, and once you've found it stick to it, and never be tempted to try something different, especially on race day.

TOILET TROUBLES ... NOT 'DOING A PAULA'

The wittily named Runners' Trots are characterized by a sudden and impossible-to-ignore need to get to a toilet while running. Don't think you're alone in either worrying about them or suffering from them, as it's something that can afflict even top runners. Who can forget Paula Radcliffe's famous and very public moment on the Embankment during her record-breaking London Marathon win? Running plays merry havoc with your digestion, jostling your intestines and reducing blood flow to them. On top of this you'll be chucking sugary gels and fluids down your throat, so is it any wonder that occasionally your bowels rebel? Dehydration makes the problem even worse, so longer runs in warm weather can be especially bad news.

If Runners' Trots are plaguing your running, the first thing to do is to investigate your personal transit time. Eat some sweetcorn and simply see how long it takes to re-emerge. Exercise will speed up your transit time significantly, so this also needs to be factored in. Once you have an idea of your transit time and daily bowel habits, you can plan your running around it. Refer to your food diary, and see if any particular foods correspond to bad bouts of the trots. Likely suspects are energy gels, excessive amounts of fibrous food, tea, coffee, spicy or fatty food, alcohol or high doses of Vitamin C. If you happen to be intolerant to gluten or dairy, then either of these food groups can also cause a reaction. Cut out any foods that you know you react badly to, and try to time your training so that it is sympathetic to your body's transit time. Keeping yourself hydrated on long runs is key to keeping the trots at bay, so practising taking fluids on board little and often right from the start of your runs is essential.

A good tip for morning runners that I use is to get up a bit earlier, have a tea or coffee to get things moving, pay a visit to the loo once the drink has kicked in, and then head out to run. For interval and tempo sessions, take advantage of the stimulating effect of exercise by having a warm-up loop that brings you back home for a pitstop before you start trying to run hard. Plan routes that have available toilet stops – supermarkets are great – and it never hurts to have a few sheets of toilet paper or wipes in your bum bag. Choose foods that tend to be naturally constipating on days when you've got runs planned. White bread/bagels, white rice or pasta will all do the job.

If all this fails to bring the problem under control, I'd strongly recommend consulting a doctor to check that there's no underlying issue such as IBS (Irritable Bowel Syndrome) or food allergies contributing to the problem. Do not start popping blockers such as Imodium without your doctor's say-so; although they can be a race saver on marathon day they should not be used as a matter of course or as a just in case preventative.

Training through the Winter: the Unpleasant Reality of a Spring Marathon

Most major marathons take place in either the spring or autumn to offer both elite and recreational runners the best chance of decent running conditions. Unfortunately, if you opt for a spring marathon such as London, Paris or Rotterdam you'll be doing the bulk of your training and your longest runs through the worst of the winter. Your strength work and swimming should be totally unaffected, unless you end up completely snowed in, but keeping your running going can be a tougher proposition.

CLOTHING
In Level 1 I covered the principles of layering and how, with modern technical clothing, you can stay dry and warm no matter how foul the weather. With a quality wicking base layer, preferably merino wool or silk, a lightweight

insulating fleece mid-layer and a weatherproof shell, you can run in almost any conditions. I raced in a 120-mile ultra in the Canadian Arctic in temperatures as low as -40 °C wearing this combination with an extra insulating layer, and as long as I was moving I was comfortable. Getting out of the door on a cold and dark winter's day is the hardest bit, but as long as you've thought about your kit, once you get going it's never so bad. Remember, no matter how tempting it is, don't wrap up too warm or you'll be stopping to strip off after 10 minutes. You want to be slightly cool leaving the house. A little trick I use to give me a morale-boosting lift is to warm my hat, gloves and socks on a radiator. Just that little bit of toasty warmth on these extremities can make all the difference and won't make you overheat. Don't forget that wearing a hat and gloves can make a massive difference to staying warm. A full beanie can often be too warm, though, so, take a tip from cross-country skiers and try an insulating headband that'll keep your ears warm while allowing your head to breathe. Another great option for your head is a Buff: a simple tube of stretchy material, this can be a beanie (for cold conditions), headband or scarf, and it's well worth having one in your bum bag. With cold rain or snow, it's often your feet that suffer. It's possible to get running shoes, especially trail shoes, that are waterproof, but I've never found them to be particularly effective. Tread in a puddle that comes over your ankle and they're equally good at keeping water in, and become your own mobile paddling pools. Waterproof socks such as SealSkinz provide an effective solution for keeping your feet warm and dry, and even come in a luxurious merino wool-lined version.

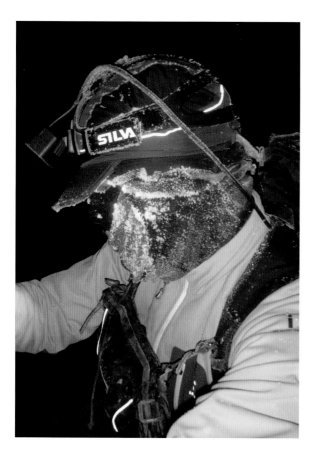

Even at -40 °C and in the dark, you can still go running

On the subject of wet feet, there are few things more demoralizing before you even start running than putting on cold, wet shoes. The traditional method of stuffing them with newspaper and leaving them near, but never on, a radiator works well, but you can now get purpose-designed shoe dryers called Dampires that are simple to use and reuse.

SAFETY CONCERNS

The biggest danger to runners during the winter months is cars not seeing you in the rain or low light. The best advice is to get off the roads whenever possible. Unlit country lanes are absolute deathtraps, and you're far better off braving a bit of mud and finding a footpath route. Failing that, or in town, do everything to get yourself seen. Most running clothing and shoes have reflective piping, but a hi-viz tabard is an essential piece of kit for winter road runners. You can also get hi-viz gloves and hats. The gloves in particular, because they're moving, can be especially visible. Clipping a rear bike light or two to your bum bag is an excellent idea, and you can get some really compact and light ones. A head torch will not only help you to see pot-holes and kerbs on unlit roads, but can make a real difference to oncoming traffic seeing you. There are plenty of lightweight models available from brands such as Silva and Petzl, and for road running where the priority is being seen you only need to spend £30–£50. If you want to head off-road in the dark, which is probably one of my favourite types of running, you'll need a head torch with a bit more power. Seek advice from a specialist off-road running shop such as Pete Bland Sports, but expect to pay £150 or more. Again, if there is snow and ice on the ground, getting off treacherous roads and pavements and hitting the trails is by far the most sensible option. Running off-road in snow is a great workout and elicits almost childlike joy in me. If you're forced to stick to tarmac, you can get excellent pull-on snow studs for your running shoes called Get-a-Grips. The carbide studs make a real difference on ice or compacted snow, and on patches of uncovered road you can't feel them through your shoes. Don't leave ordering a set until the big freeze, as they always sell out. It's sensible to always let someone know when you're heading out to run, roughly where you're going and how long you plan to be. In winter this advice is even more pertinent, and always take a mobile phone with you.

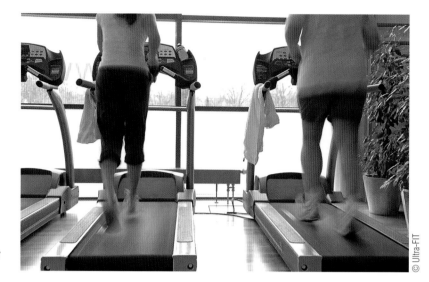

Treadmills, only for when running outside is completely impossible

© Ultra-FIT

INDOOR OPTIONS

Running indoors on a treadmill should be avoided in all but the most inclement weather. Apart from the skull-crushing tedium of plodding away in the gym, running on a treadmill is a very poor approximation of real running, and encourages the development of bad running technique. A key part of the running stride is bringing your leg back and through, and on a treadmill this is done for you by the belt. You're very cramped, and even shorter runners won't have a natural stride length on a treadmill. Finally, every stride you take is exactly the same, which increases the likelihood of developing an overuse injury. The odd session on a treadmill if you really can't face heading out is okay, but don't let it become a habit. Set the treadmill to a one per cent gradient to give a more realistic simulation of running outdoors, and make sure you have plenty of fluids to hand. Kit and clothing is so good now, though, that only absolutely atrocious weather should force you indoors and on to a treadmill.

You might well already be completing your cycling workouts indoors on an exercise bike, in a spinning class or on a turbo trainer, and even if you've been riding outdoors during the summer and autumn, heading indoors through the worst of the winter can be sensible. With the right kit, though, cycling outdoors is still possible on all but the iciest and snowiest days, and mountain biking in the snow is hard to beat for its grin factor.

WINTER BLUES AND MAINTAINING MOTIVATION

As well as the serious and debilitating clinical condition SAD (Seasonal Affective Disorder), many of us suffer from a dip in mood and motivation during the short winter days. As this dip in mood is thought to be caused by a drop in the brain's 'happy chemical', serotonin, the good news for runners is that exercise causes serotonin to be released, and can help counter the condition. It's easy to get caught in a vicious circle of not having the motivation to run and then getting even more blue. Try to get at least a few of your runs each week done during daylight by using lunch breaks, or running during the middle of the day at weekends. Remove every possible obstruction to getting out running, as even the smallest blip, such as a misplaced glove, can be enough for you to ditch the session. If you're running in the morning, or when you get home from work, make sure all your kit is laid out, ordered and ready to go. Make 'training dates' with running friends, or report your training on Facebook or other social media. Knowing someone is waiting to run with you, or that your friends are following your training, are both great for motivation. If you run in the morning, think about investing in a dawn-simulating alarm clock, which uses a daylight bulb coming on gradually to wake you. I've used one from Lumie for the last couple of winters and have found it has made a massive difference.

Sunrise simulating alarm clock, great for those winter early starts

You wake up feeling refreshed and ready to go, rather than the shocked and fuzzy sensation waking to a regular alarm in the dark gives you. Think about booking some warm weather training to give you a bit of sun, a boost and something to look forward to. There are many companies offering bespoke running packages, or simply find somewhere pleasantly warm, get a group of running mates together and just head off.

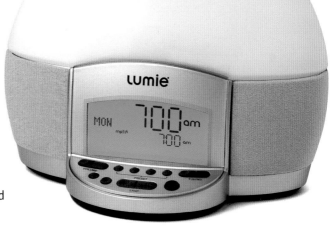

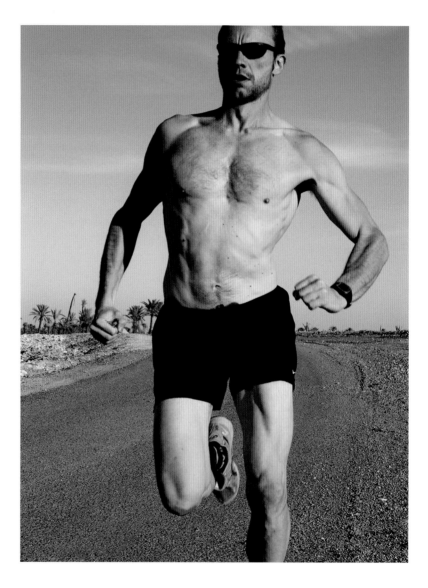

The author winter training in Morocco

Club La Santa on Lanzarote is geared specifically towards sports training and has a brilliant climate for running through the whole winter. Finally, to reward all the hard work you're putting in, promise yourself some little treats for completing all your training sessions. A meal at your favourite restaurant, a long luxurious bath or a massage can all be perfect carrots to keep you going.

The Plan

	Week 13	Week 14	Week 15	Week 16	Week 17	Week 18	Week 19	Week 20
Monday	Recovery session. Yoga/Pilates or rest	Recovery session. Yoga/Pilates or rest	Recovery session. Yoga/Pilates or rest	Recovery session. Yoga/Pilates or rest	Recovery session. Yoga/Pilates or rest	Recovery session. Yoga/Pilates or rest	Recovery session. Yoga/Pilates or rest	Recovery session. Yoga/Pilates or rest
Tuesday	Run 1: 30 mins tempo (10–**15**–5) Followed by strength routine	Run 1: 32 mins tempo (10–**17**–5) Followed by strength routine	Run 1: 35 mins tempo (10–**20**–5) Followed by strength routine	Run 1: 37 mins tempo (10–**22**–5) Followed by strength routine	Run 1: 40 mins tempo (10–**25**–5) Followed by strength routine	Run 1: 42 mins tempo (10–**27**–5) Followed by strength routine	Run 1: 45 mins tempo (10–**30**–5) Followed by strength routine	Run 1: 25 mins tempo (10–**5**–5) Followed by strength routine
Wednesday	30 mins swim	30 mins swim	30 mins swim	30 mins swim	30 mins swim	30 mins swim	30 mins swim	30 mins swim
Thursday	Run 2: Intervals 2 x 4 mins (3 mins reco) Followed by strength routine	Run 2: Intervals 3 x 4 mins (3 mins reco) Followed by strength routine	Run 2: Intervals 3 x 5 mins (4 mins reco) Followed by strength routine	Run 2: Intervals 4 x 5 mins (4 mins reco) Followed by strength routine	Run 1: Intervals 5 x 5 mins (4 mins reco) Followed by strength routine	Run 1: Intervals 6 x 4 mins (4 mins reco) Followed by strength routine	Run 2: Intervals 6 x 5 mins (4 mins reco) Followed by strength routine	Run 2: Intervals 10 x 1 min (1 min reco) Followed by long stretch massage
Friday	Rest day	Rest day	Rest day	Rest day	Rest day	Rest day	Rest day	Rest day
Saturday	2–3 hours hike	Run 3: LSD 60 mins	Run 3: LSD 70 mins	Run 3: LSD 80 mins	Run 3: LSD 90 mins	Run 3: LSD 100 mins	Run 3: LSD 110 mins	Day before easy-paced 20 mins jog in race kit
Sunday	Cycle 60 mins	Cycle 65 mins	Cycle 70 mins	Cycle 80 mins	Cycle 90 mins	Cycle 90 mins	Cycle 90 mins	Half marathon race or run

The Sessions

MONDAY

This stays as a rest or recovery day. With longer weekend runs and rides during this build-up to a half marathon, it's essential that you listen to your body and are honest with yourself. If you wake up on Monday morning feeling even the slightest bit fatigued, take a complete rest day, or make any activity extremely gentle. The quality of the three running sessions is the most important aspect of your training, and if you're starting the week tired, that'll be compromised. Try to pack too much in and you'll be reducing your fitness gains and increasing your risk of injury.

TUESDAY

This stays as a tempo session followed by the strength routine. You'll be building the duration of your tempo run until, by the end of the level, it'll be up to 30 minutes. If you've made the switch to heart rate training, you'll be looking to run the tempo time in Zone 3. Don't be surprised if this is a slower pace than you were running your tempo at when using perceived exertion. Stick to the heart rate zones: they're tested, accurate, and will make sure you're running at the correct pace.

WEDNESDAY

This is a day for the pool. If you're struggling to fit in your strength routine after your Tuesday and Thursday run sessions, at this stage in the plan you can drop to one strength session and can use Wednesdays for it. You won't necessarily continue to gain functional strength, but you will maintain the excellent base you've already laid. Follow the strength routine with your pool session and your legs will be fine for Thursday's session.

THURSDAY

These interval sessions are probably the toughest workout of the week, but if completed correctly and at the right intensity they deliver the most signficant fitness gains. Really focus on running hard and strong, and pacing the intervals evenly. Using a heart rate monitor makes this much easier. Aim for mid-Zone 3 pushing into Zone 4 for the work intervals. Don't go off too hard in an attempt to kick your heart rate up too quickly. Look for a consistent pace that allows your heart rate to build strongly, hitting the target zone after 30–60 seconds.

FRIDAY

No ifs, no buts: this is a rest day. You've got a tough weekend coming, so make the most of it.

SATURDAY

We start the level with a long hike to bring in some variety and a change of scenery, and to show you that you can do two to three hours on your feet. Go somewhere scenic and hilly, and enjoy the break from running. For the rest of the level, Saturdays are all about LSD, building your endurance, practising your eating and drinking on the go, and making sure that your kit is spot on. By the end of this level all of these variables should be set in stone and almost second nature to you.

SUNDAY

We build your Sunday ride up to 90 minutes during this block, so if you're riding indoors I hope you've got some good playlists to listen to or DVDs to watch. Ride how you feel. It's likely that your legs will feel heavy from Saturday's run for the first 30 minutes or so, but when they loosen up, push a bit harder and get your heart and lungs working hard. You've got a rest day on Monday, so you can afford to really tire yourself out.

CHAPTER 4

Level 4: Weeks 21–28

Introduction

With a half marathon under your belt, you're in the home straight and making the final push towards the full 26.2 miles. You should be full of confidence, but even more so than ever, now's the time to stick to the plan, be disciplined about your running intensity, and keep your training balanced. It's during this period, when runners are stepping up from half to full marathon, that injury rates typically soar.

In most traditional marathon plans, the overwhelming focus is on four to six mega-long three- to four-hour weekend runs. With another three or four running sessions on top of this scheduled during the week, it's no wonder that runners following these plans get injured, ill and demotivated. The argument is that these long runs prepare you physically and mentally for the demands of marathon day. If you can get through them without injury or illness, and if they don't leave you hobbling through your other training sessions, this might be the case, but they're two major ifs. By adopting an approach where you still do long, but not excessively long, weekend runs and incorporate cross-training workouts, you'll still develop that essential endurance but won't trash yourself. This'll allow you to train consistently through the whole week, rather than spending the first few days of it shattered. It'll ensure that your other training sessions are high quality, and significantly lower your chance of injury and overtraining. Even though your longest training run will 'only' be two and a half hours, you'll have the strength and fitness to cope with the extra one to two hours that marathon day will involve. Most importantly, though, you won't be injured. Don't worry that you won't have run especially close to the actual race distance: it's not essential for race day success. When I was training for a 120-mile race in the Canadian Arctic which I hoped to complete in 40–50 hours, my longest training runs were eight to 10 hours. If I'd gone out at the weekends and tried to be on my feet for 20–30 hours, my body would have been in pieces for the rest of the week and I wouldn't have got any other training done. With shorter weekend efforts, though, I was able to recover quickly and train consistently through the whole week. That consistency for six months gave me the bulk of my fitness, rather than the weekend runs, and I went on to win the race in 38:59, setting a new course record. Stick to your guns, stick to the plan and don't be tempted to run longer. You might have friends who are following traditional plans and heading out for those three- to four-hour runs, but don't be psyched out by this. You're doing plenty of other training that they're not, and I can guarantee you'll be fitter, stronger and healthier than them when you get to the start line.

HOW FAST CAN I EXPECT TO RUN?

One of the commonest mistakes many first time marathoners make is to wildly underestimate how long a marathon will take them to complete. Many runners randomly conjure a figure out of the air because that's what their mate ran or because they reckon, as a 'real runner', they should be able to break, say, four hours. Doing this not only piles unnecessary and unrealistic pressure on you but sets you up for a likely pacing disaster on the day. Going off too fast, with an unrealistic goal in mind, is probably one of the worst things you can do, can easily ruin your whole day, and can put all that hard training to waste. The best way to approach race day, for a first timer, is not to have a hard and fast time goal in mind, and certainly not to make it public knowledge. Your goals should simply be to enjoy it, get round feeling good and run a consistent race. For the sake of pacing and giving your supporters an idea of when you're likely to be at certain points of the race, making a calculation based on your half marathon performance can give a reasonably accurate range.

It's not just a case of doubling your half marathon time, although it's amazing how many people do this. A good rule of thumb for a first timer is to take your half marathon time, double it and then add a range of 10–20 per cent on top of that. So, if you've managed a two-hour half marathon, a realistic target range would be 4:24–4:48 for the full marathon. Don't immediately fixate on the lower figure: that's your best case scenario with everything going to plan. Somewhere bang in the middle of the range is a far more likely outcome. For a realistic shot at a sub four-hour marathon – a standard many people set for themselves – you'll have needed to have run a half marathon in around 1:45, and even then you'll still have to have a really good day.

If you're not happy with the predicted time this formula gives you for your marathon, don't ignore it and stubbornly try to run the time you think you're capable of. You'll have a disastrous day. I've seen it so many times, mostly from overcompetitive guys, and you'll probably end up injured and completing the course slower than your predicted time after hobbling the last eight to 10 miles. Either swallow your pride, be realistic and run to the level you're really capable of, or consider postponing your marathon debut until your half marathon fitness predicts a time that you consider acceptable. Repeat Level 3 to improve your half marathon time if you must, but simply completing a marathon, running consistently and strongly throughout, is a massive achievement irrespective of time. Leave your ego at home, run to your predicted ability and save chasing the clock until you've got a couple of marathons under your belt and you genuinely know what you're capable of.

A final note on predicted times. Many bigger marathons ask you to predict your time so that you can be zoned at the start with runners of equal ability. Please be honest, be realistic and don't bump yourself up so that you get across the start line quicker. It's selfish to put yourself in too fast a zone, and you'll be unnecessarily forcing faster runners to dodge round you and slowing them down. Almost all big marathons now have personalized timing chips, so getting across the start line quicker isn't an issue, and no matter how long it takes you'll still get your genuine time.

HOW DO I PACE MY MARATHON?

Once you have your realistic predicted time range, you'll be aiming initially for a time bang in the middle, but how do you pace this?

Many GPS-style watches can display speed and pace. However, although their accuracy and satellite acquisition have improved massively, the pace they display can be a bit uneven, and they can be badly affected by tall buildings on city centre courses.

If you've been using heart rate in training, it's possible to carry this method through to race day and aim to sit in low to mid-Zone 2. However, with race day nerves and excitement, heart rate can be inaccurate, and although it can be good to use through the mid-section of the race once you've settled down, it can be all over the place early on.

Another option is to go back to basics and to run on perceived effort and feel. Reconnect with that Level 6 running pace that we learnt at the beginning of the plan. There'll be plenty of people around to check that you can still chat, although they might not all be that responsive. You should feel as if you're consciously holding back and that your pace is noticeably slow, especially during the first 15–20 miles.

Many of the larger marathons have pacers running the course, and if your target zone corresponds to one of the pace groups on offer then following the pacer is a great way to stay on track. The pacers are usually experienced marathoners who'll be pacing a time significantly slower than their own personal best. This allows them to run comfortably and concentrate on ensuring a perfectly even and accurate pace. Having personally paced the London Marathon three times (the 3:30 group), you certainly feel a weight of expectation from the runners following you, and looking back at the throng behind you on the Embankment is truly amazing. It's just a shame that everyone comes streaming past on the Mall, leaving the poor pacers to finish seemingly on their own, 10 seconds or so under their specified time.

Almost all marathons will be mile-marked, and a simple pacing table is still, I believe, the best way to pace your race. Work out your mile splits for your fastest, mid-range and slowest predicted times. Produce a small, laminated, credit card sized table that you can easily attach to your wrist next to your watch with an elastic band to show you the times you should be passing through every mile at. Run the first couple of miles on feel and then, once the crowds have thinned a bit and you've settled into a rhythm, see how you're going compared with your table when you pass mile three. You'll know whether you need to ease down or speed up, and where in your range you're running. It'll give you something to focus on every mile, provide a valuable distraction and, even if you're planning on following a pacer, monitoring and being aware of your own pace is essential, as there's no guarantee how good they are or even if they'll make the full distance: pacers have off days too. It's also a really good idea to print off a few copies for your supporters, as it'll give them a guide when to expect you at viewing points and the finish.

WHY A HALF MARATHON ISN'T HALF A MARATHON

For absolute distance, obviously 13.1 miles is half of 26.2 miles. However, for the impact on your physiology and physical effort, 26.2 miles is so much more than double 13.1 miles. I'm not trying to scare you, belittle your fantastic achievement of running a half marathon, or put you off attempting to run the full distance. All I'm trying to do is to ensure you have enough respect for the distance and are pre-armed with the knowledge needed for a successful race day. The oft-used expression is that 20 miles is the halfway point in a marathon, and in my experience this is about right. The final six miles doesn't have to be a hellish suffer-fest, but if you've overcooked your pace early on, or have failed to eat and drink consistently, it easily can be. If you feel as if you're working hard going through 13 miles, don't fool yourself into thinking, 'I'm halfway, I can tough it out': you can't and you won't. Back off then to a realistic and sensible pace and you might just salvage your race. Conservative and sensible pacing up to 20 miles is the only recipe for success, and unless you heed this advice you won't run a good marathon. I'm not trying to sound overly dramatic, but with the massive number of people completing marathons every year, as an achievement it's become wrongly devalued. Not training, trying to run too fast, staggering round in little above walking pace and then not being able to walk for days afterwards is unnecessary, is not running a marathon and, if you've followed this plan, not what you'll be doing.

WHAT IS THE WALL, AND DOES IT EXIST?

Everybody has heard horror stories about the Wall: an infamous point 18–22 miles into a marathon where your legs suddenly stop moving and you're reduced to a crawl. You'll hear supposed experts saying it's the point where your body attempts to make the switch to inefficient fat-burning, but for most people who think they've hit the Wall it's nothing to do with this and is totally avoidable. Many people take part in ultra marathons that are further than 26.2 miles, and often over 100 miles, and they manage these without hitting any 'walls'. Almost every aspirant marathon runner who has claimed to have had their race day scuppered by the Wall has actually done one of the following:

Too fast too early: Being too ambitious about target time, and running too fast for your ability, is the number one reason behind a horrible final six to eight miles. You know from your training and your half marathon what you're capable of, and although race day might give you a slight boost, it won't make you a superman.

Not enough training: Consistency through this final eight-week block is essential, and any missed sessions or compromised weeks will come back to bite you. Complete the plan, pace yourself correctly, and you will run a great marathon. There will always be people who claim to have run marathons on little or no training, but it won't have been enjoyable, they will have slowed massively in the last six to eight miles, and they won't have walked normally for at least a week afterwards.

Not eating: I've already stressed the importance of fuelling little and often right from the start of any long run, and from your training you'll know exactly what and when you eat on marathon day. Fail to eat from the start, or neglect regular top-ups, and you'll simply run out of fuel.

Not drinking: The biggest cause of supposed Wall casualties is becoming dehydrated, but as long as you drink according to your physiology and the weather conditions, this is completely avoidable.

Keeping Mentally Strong

You only have to watch an elite marathon runner to see how important focus, concentration and a positive psychological approach are to successful distance running. Over the course of training for and running a marathon you'll go through the complete gamut of emotions: abject misery at the beginning of a midwinter training run, contrasting with the incredibly smug satisfaction and virtuous glow once you've finished it; almost crippling nerves the night before a race; and then the relief and elation when you cross the finishing line. Having got to this stage in the plan you'll have already overcome significant psychological hurdles, shown true mental grit getting through long training runs, and displayed awesome levels of self-motivation and determination. However, in the final weeks before your marathon, I can almost guarantee that doubts will start to creep into your mind, and you'll start to question whether you're really up to the task. These doubts are perfectly normal, and a few pre-race nerves are beneficial to a good performance. It's important not to let them get on top of you, though, and to affect your final preparations and performance negatively on race day. Knowing how to keep yourself up, how to give yourself a bit of a pep talk, what to expect as race day looms, and keeping your brain in check from start line to finish, are all just as important as those final physical preparations.

TALK TO THE CHIMP

Dr Steve Peters, a brilliant sports psychiatrist who's worked wonders with members of the British cycling team, including Victoria Pendleton, Bradley Wiggins and Sir Chris Hoy, uses the analogy of an annoying chimpanzee. The chimp will chatter away at you, reminding you of all your doubts, fears, worries and insecurities. Many of those doubts, such as the weather on race day, you have no control over, and worrying about them is simply wasted energy. Many people try to shut the chimp up by ignoring him and locking him in a box, but he's a persistent and loud primate and will make himself heard. Even if you try to ignore him, his cries and chattering will pop into your head throughout the day and eat away at your energy and confidence. The solution is to make an appointment every day with your chimp, let him out of his box and calmly address all of the nagging doubts he raises. If it's a doubt you have control over, such as getting to the start on time, take positive steps to do everything you can to dispel it. If it's something you have no control over, such as the weather or what people will think if you fail, accept that there's nothing you can do and move on. Eventually, by spending five to 10 minutes each day talking to your chimp, he'll shut up and stay quietly in his box. It might seem a bit weird, but having met Steve and several of his charges, I'm a convert and, if necessary, I converse with my chimp when out for my morning runs. Especially in the weeks before a big race, I've found it an invaluable process in keeping my nerves in check, maintaining a positive frame of mind and getting to the start line with complete confidence in my preparation and ability. Try it and shut that chimp up.

HAVE CONFIDENCE IN YOUR TRAINING

The most important thing to remember is the 28-plus weeks of consistent training you've put in to get you to the start line. You're functionally strong for running, have developed fantastic endurance, have great running technique and, most importantly, you're injury free. If you're having any doubts, have a look back through your training diary and remind yourself of the progress you've made. Having followed this plan, the main niggling doubt will be that, compared with more traditional plans, you won't have done enough running. Remind yourself of the following:

All of your running has been focused: You've accumulated no meaningless junk miles and have optimized every workout by ensuring you've worked at exactly the right intensity.

You've done so much more than just run: For every extra workout that your marathon peers have spent mindlessly pounding the pavements, you've spent time strengthening your body with specifically designed exercises, you've optimized your recovery to maximize fitness gains, and you've incorporated cross-training to gain robust fitness without increasing injury risk.

Kit, nutrition and pacing have all been practised: Every aspect of race day has been rehearsed in training, and any mistakes have been made already and rectified. Stick to what you've tried and tested in training and race day will go smoothly. Don't stress the extra distance: remember, the extra 60–90 minutes that many plans would have heaped on top of your long runs still wouldn't have taken you to 26.2 miles, would have made you more to prone to injury, and would have compromised your other training sessions. Every first-timer on the start line will be running to a certain extent into the unknown, but you will be doing so strong, uninjured and perfectly prepared.

WHAT TO EXPECT ON RACE DAY

If you're running a big city centre marathon then you can expect an atmosphere unlike any other you've experienced. This'll start at the Race Expo and

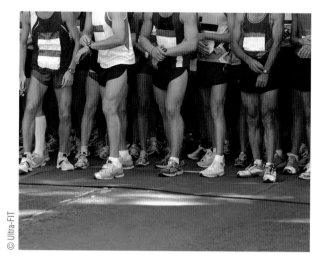

Waiting for the gun

registration, where the reality of what you're about to do will really kick in. The venue will be charged with the nerves of thousands of runners, and it's far too easy to get caught up in it and overwhelmed. The golden rule is to stand firm, have confidence in your preparation and race day plans, and not to get swayed by all the shiny toys, stands and kit into making any last-minute changes. The nerve level cranks up another notch if there's a pre-race pasta party, and up again travelling to the race start. Don't get sucked into conversations about what kit you're using or what training you've done. You're not going to change any of your race day plans and you certainly can't change the training you've done. People will want to talk about these things because they're nervous and want affirmation that what they've done is enough and that their plans for the day are correct. Be polite, but keep focused on your own race, keep reminding yourself about the excellent preparation you've done, and stay calm. At the start you'll see all sorts of warming-up, stretching and nervous pacing going on. You'll also see the longest toilet queues you've ever seen. Again, keep focused on your own race and plans. You didn't bounce around and stretch before your long training runs, so don't start doing it now. Go for a light jog or walk to get away from the crowds and find some head space, but make sure you know exactly where you need to be for the start and how long it'll take to get there. You don't want a last-minute rush and to be pumped full of adrenalin as you set off. Be early, be calm and be focused.

At the gun, be prepared for a temporary massive sense of relief that you're finally off, and then a huge surge of adrenalin. You need to rein this in, though, and stay in control. If it's a big race, you won't have any choice about taking things steady, but don't panic about crossing the start line quickly or trying to dodge round people. Just take it easy, and remember that your timing chip won't start until you cross the start line and that weaving around slower runners adds distance and wastes energy. Be patient and even at the biggest races you'll be running relatively freely and obstruction free within a mile.

Then it's a case of relaxing into your planned pace and soaking up the amazing atmosphere from the crowd. Many runners claim that the crowd support at a big city centre event is the equivalent of at least a 10-mile boost. I'd certainly go along with this, and partaking and interacting with the carnival atmosphere will literally make the miles fly by. Soak it all up and totally immerse yourself in the party atmosphere on the route. This is why I can't understand runners who shut themselves off from the crowd by plugging straight into an MP3 player. They're missing out on one of the best legal performance-enhancers available, one that can easily carry you through the first 15–20 miles almost effortlessly.

The joy of crossing the line

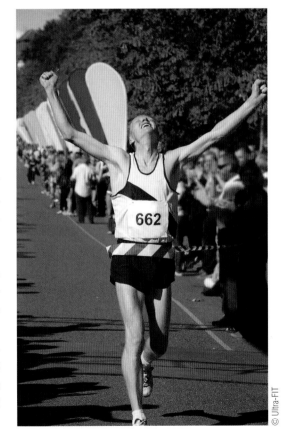

Eventually, though, the effort and duration of what you're doing will catch up with you. With good pacing and fuelling, this shouldn't be too bad or too early on, but you will have to dig in, focus and concentrate. Rather than drawing from the crowd, turn your focus inwards and draw on your own inner strength. Remind yourself of the training you've done, the sacrifices you've made, the friends and family who've supported you, and just how good crossing that finish line will be. If it works for you, now's the time to plug into that MP3 player and that great playlist of motivational tracks. Concentrate on your pacing. Hopefully you should be in single-figure miles left at this stage and can count them off one by one on your pacing sheet. Keep talking to yourself, and don't be afraid to give yourself a bit of a ticking off if your drive starts to waver. Count foot strikes – one of Paula Radcliffe's favourite tricks – or even have a small picture of a loved one on the back of your pacing card to draw inspiration from.

With one or two miles to go, it's time to come out of your private world and embrace the crowd again. You've put so much work in to get to this stage that you deserve to enjoy it. As you go under the 25-mile banner I can guarantee that, no matter how tired you're feeling, you'll find some extra strength and be able to pick up your pace. High-five the crowd, congratulate runners around you and let the euphoria of the moment wash away any pain. Have a smile to yourself as you pass through 26 miles, and silently curse the Royal Family for the extra 0.2 miles, but once round an athletics track and you're done.

Expect equal measures of relief and elation on crossing the finish line and maybe even a little hint of sadness that such an amazing experience is over. You'll mutter the classic line 'never again', but as your finisher's medal is placed round your neck the pain is replaced by pride you can finally say, 'I'm a marathon runner'.

24 Hours to Go: a Practical Guide

WHAT TO EAT AND DRINK, AND WHEN

In Level 3 we've covered when and what to eat before long training runs and races, and there's no need to do anything different in the days before your marathon. There's certainly no need to eat vast amounts of pasta or to 'carb load'. Two to three days before your marathon, start to ease back on foods high in fibre, and avoid heavy and hard to digest fats and proteins.

You'll have already discovered during your training what meal works best for you the night before a long run, so stick with it. If your marathon is abroad, check to see what types of food are on offer at your hotel, or what restaurants are nearby. I'm a big fan of exploring local cuisines when I travel, but the night before a big race is not the time for it. When I took part in the Powerman Malaysia duathlon, I don't think the tiny Italian restaurant in the small town of Perak knew what'd hit it when hundreds of athletes wanting their pre-race pasta and pizza hit suddenly turned up on their doorstep.

The day and night before your marathon, probably one of the most important nutritional factors is keeping hydrated. You don't want to be having to drink loads on the morning of the race, so making sure your body is fully hydrated the day and night before is really important. Have a water bottle to hand at all times during the 24 hours before the race, and just keep sipping. This is especially important when you're travelling, or walking round the Expo. Keep the water going in along with some electrolyte salts. You might end up having to go to the loo a couple of times during the night, but you'll probably have a restless night because of nerves anyway.

On the morning of the race, again, treat it exactly the same as your long training runs, and stick to your routine. Make sure you allow at least two hours between your breakfast and the starter's gun. Eat whatever works for you, but again avoiding fibre, fats and heavy protein. Pre-marathon, I'll go for two poached eggs on two bagels, a decent cup of coffee and 500 ml of carbohy-drate sports drink. I'll then take a 250 ml bottle of water with me to sip on the way to and at the start. With the fluids you drank the day before, this should leave you perfectly hydrated but not needing the loo within minutes of the start. If you're having to travel on race morning and will be leaving home or where you're staying more than two hours before the race is due to start, have your breakfast as normal, and have an energy bar or similar on hand to top up your energy levels two hours before the off. Also, for every extra hour on top of the two, take an additional 100 ml of water to sip.

Once the gun goes off, it's time to implement that fuelling and drinking strategy you've developed in training. Remember the maxim of eating and drinking little and often from the gun and continuing all the way through the race. If you've trained using a sports drink that isn't supplied at the aid stations, carry your own supply in the bum bag/rucksack water bladder/bottle system you've been using. The initial extra weight will not adversely affect your performance, as you're used to running with it in training, it'll get lighter as you drink it, you'll be totally confident you'll get all the fluids you need, and you'll be able to pass by the drinks stations scrums. If you're just running on plain water and relying on gels and solid food for your energy, use the same system to carry them as you did in training. A neat trick on race day, though, is to find out the brand of mineral water on offer at the drinks stations and buy a sports-style bottle from the same manufacturer. You can then just put the sports cap on the open bottles dished out, save the water from splashing all over the place and be able to drink in a steady and quantifiable way, rather than having to gulp hurriedly from an opened bottle.

WHERE TO STAY

You should try to make life as easy and stress-free for yourself as possible on marathon day. If you don't live locally to the race or have friends or family who live nearby, finding a hotel close to the start line and confirming a booking early is one of the best things you can possibly do to facilitate this. Check when you book that they'll do breakfast early enough for you on race day, and how long it'll take you to get to the start. In an ideal world, for a Sunday marathon, I'd take the Friday and Monday off work and book a room for Friday, Saturday and Sunday night. This would allow me to attend registration and the Expo on the Friday, avoiding both the crowds and the collective panic on the Saturday. You can then have a super-chilled day on the Saturday, get your 20-minute leg-loosening run done, and make sure all your kit and equipment is ready to go. Use Saturday to also confirm how you're going to get from the finish back to your hotel. Remember, there might be significant road closures and large crowds of spectators and competitors on public transport. Taking the Monday off work may seem excessive, but I promise you you'll be grateful of it. Not having to spend Sunday post-run stuck cramping in a car or train, but instead relaxing in a hotel bath or pool, is the least you deserve, and you won't be at your productive best on Monday morning anyway.

NOT SLEEPING

Pre-race nerves, fretting about not waking up and missing the start, all the water you've drunk, a strange bed, and sudden panics that you've forgotten your safety pins, can all mean that you don't get a great night's sleep before your marathon. This happens to almost everyone, but the good news is that one night of poor sleep has very little, if any, affect on physical performance the following day. You might feel a little groggy, but it won't stop you running 26.2 miles to the best of your abilities. Don't stress about trying to get to bed or sleep too early, and if you're lying there not sleeping and worrying, get up and watch TV, have a hot bath or even go through your race kit and checklist to reassure yourself.

ON THE START LINE

Find the lorries that take your post-run kit bag to the finish, and get your bag stowed. Put a full change of clean and dry kit in this bag, including socks and compression tights if you use them, and a small towel for wiping yourself down. Think about what you always tend to crave to eat after your long runs – in my case a millionaire's shortbread – and if practical stash some of it. Having pounded in your running shoes for 26.2 miles, a pair of comfy flip-flops to put on are absolute bliss. Many people leave handing their kit over to the very last minute so they can keep their warm clothes on, but you'll just be setting yourself up for unnecessary queuing and stress. Take a spare old sweatshirt or fleece that you don't mind ditching and, if rain is forecast, an old bin-bag with a hole cut for your head is hard to beat. Another stay-dry option is one of the disposable plastic ponchos you get at theme parks. Join the toilet queues early, and take a few sheets of toilet paper with you, as it always runs out. Make your way to the starting pens with plenty of time to spare, and if you're planning on running with a pacer and they're provided, find the correct one for your target time. Wait for the last possible moment before ditching your disposable layers, and enjoy the run.

FRIENDS AND SUPPORTERS
Having friends, family and supporters on the course can give you a massive boost. There's no point, though, in them dashing around trying to get to numerous spectator spots, missing you at them all, and then being late for you at the finish. Having supported my wife on two London marathons, it's a far more stressful day than running it. Realistically, ask them to get to a couple of spots on the route and, most importantly, the finish. An early spot within the first six miles, later on at 15–18 miles when it might be getting tough, and then at the finish is an ideal spread. Give them a copy of your pacing card so they'll know when to expect you, but stress the importance of them not hanging around on the course waiting for you, especially at the last spectating point. It's really easy for them to miss you, and the most important place for them to be is at the finish. When I was pacing the London Marathon one year, despite me being bang on pace, carrying a lollipop and having a hoard of people following me, my wife still failed to spot me at two viewing points. Get your supporters to carry a banner or some bright helium balloons to stand out in the crowd, and make sure they know what you're planning to wear. At the finish, prearrange a meeting point. Mobile networks will be overloaded, and you won't have the energy or the patience to hunt for your friends. Get them

to bring some extra spare clothes, food and drink with them, in case there's been a problem with your drop bag. Ask them to sort out the easiest way to get you back to where you're staying, and although it might not seem a big deal to them to walk 800 m for a cab or bus, it could take you a very long time and you won't want to be rushed. Even if you've got your own friends and family en route, getting your name printed on your running top is an excellent way to get extra support. You'll be amazed how many people give you a shout, and it really does put an extra spring in your step.

MARATHON CHECKLISTS

Before
✓ Print name on running top
✓ Book hotel/find suitable pre- and post-race accommodation
✓ Book suitable restaurant for dinner on night before race
✓ Check hotel can do early breakfast
✓ Confirm transport route and time to start
✓ Confirm transport route from finish
✓ Confirm meeting point with supporters

Expo/registration
✓ Check time and location
✓ Photo ID and proof of entry

Start/race kit
✓ 250 ml water for pre-race
✓ Bar for pre-race if necessary
✓ Old sweatshirt/fleece
✓ Bin-bag/disposable poncho
✓ Toilet paper
✓ Race number
✓ Timing chip
✓ Safety pins
✓ Pacing card
✓ Running shoes

- ✓ Socks
- ✓ Shorts
- ✓ Running top
- ✓ Hat/gloves if cold
- ✓ Plasters for nipples
- ✓ Water bottle/hydration bladder/sports bottle cap
- ✓ Rucksack/bum bag
- ✓ Gels/bars/other race food

Finish drop bag

- ✓ Recovery drink
- ✓ Sweet and savoury snacks
- ✓ Towel
- ✓ Warm clothes
- ✓ Compression tights
- ✓ Flip-flops or comfy shoes
- ✓ Money for transport

Supporters checklist

- ✓ Confirm finish meeting point with your runner
- ✓ Confirm proposed spectating points with your runner
- ✓ Runner's pacing card
- ✓ Banner/balloons
- ✓ Spare warm clothes and food for finish

The Plan

	Week 21	Week 22	Week 23	Week 24	Week 25	Week 26	Week 27	Week 28
Monday	Recovery session. Yoga/Pilates. Swim or rest	Recovery session. Yoga/Pilates. Swim or rest	Recovery session. Yoga/Pilates. Swim or rest	Recovery session. Yoga/Pilates. Swim or rest	Recovery session. Yoga/Pilates. Swim or rest	Recovery session. Yoga/Pilates. Swim or rest	Recovery session. Yoga/Pilates. Swim or rest	Recovery session. Yoga/Pilates. Swim or rest
Tuesday	Run 1: 45 mins tempo (10–**30**–5)	Run 1: 47 mins tempo (10–**32**–5)	Run 1: 50 mins tempo (10–**35**–5)	Run 1: 52 mins tempo (10–**37**–5)	Run 1: 55 mins tempo (10–**40**–5)	Run 1: 60 mins tempo (10–**45**–5)	Run 1: 45 mins tempo (10–**30**–5)	Run 1: 25 mins tempo (10–**10**–5)
Wednesday	Strength routine	Strength routine	Strength routine	Strength routine	Strength routine	Strength routine	Strength routine	Strength routine
Thursday	Run 2: Intervals 5 x 6 mins (4 mins reco)	Run 2: Intervals 4 x 7 mins (4 mins reco)	Run 2: Intervals 4 x 8 mins (4 mins reco)	Run 2: Intervals 3 x 10 mins (4 mins reco)	Run 1: Intervals 3 x 12 mins (4 mins reco)	Run 1: Intervals 2 x 15 mins (4 mins reco)	Run 2: Intervals 5 x 4 mins (3 mins reco)	Run 2: 20 mins Easy-paced 6 x 25 m strides
Friday	Rest day	Rest day	Rest day	Rest day	Rest day	Rest day	Rest day	Rest day
Saturday	Hike 4–6 hours	Run 3: LSD 130 mins (60 mins Zone 2)	Run 3: LSD 140 mins (80 mins Zone 2)	Run 3: LSD 150 mins (100 mins Zone 2)	Run 3: LSD 150 mins (120 mins Zone 2)	Run 3: LSD 150 mins (120 mins Zone 2)	Run 3: LSD 90 mins	Day before easy-paced 20 mins jog in race kit
Sunday	Cycle 60 mins	Cycle 90 mins	Cycle 90 mins	Cycle 90 mins	Cycle 90 mins	Cycle 90 mins	Cycle 60 mins	Marathon

The Sessions

MONDAY

As through the whole plan, Monday is a rest or active recovery day to let you recover after your long weekend sessions. Through this block you'll consistently be doing up to four hours of training over the weekend, so don't be surprised if you wake up on Mondays feeling tired, sore or a bit flat. I'd strongly recommend trying to schedule in a massage on at least alternate Mondays. Personally, I find a swim session to be one of the most effective forms of active recovery, and as you're losing your Wednesday swim in this block, using Mondays to keep your swim fitness ticking over is a really good idea.

TUESDAY

Sticking with the tempo session, you'll be building up to 45 minutes of running at this pace. If you know the distance of a running loop, or have a GPS, log how far you run during the tempo block. Compare the result with the time it took you to run your first 5 km, and I reckon you'll be pretty pleased with your progress. You'll notice that the strength routine is dropped from both Tuesdays and Thursdays. This is because the length of these workouts is increasing, and fitting everything in could become difficult.

WEDNESDAY

This is now the day for your strength routine. We're dropping to one strength session per week, with the aim being to maintain the gains you've already made. Feel free to add an extra set of each exercise to the routine to make it a fuller session. Make sure you warm up before the strength work with 10 minutes of light cardiovascular exercise such as jogging, cycling, rowing or working on a cross-trainer. If you want to carry on swimming on a Wednesday, it's fine to do this after your strength workout.

THURSDAY

Through this block, the number of work intervals you'll perform in a workout drops, but their duration increases. The ideal is to be working in heart rate Zone 4, but this is a tough ask to maintain for intervals of this length. You also may find that your heart rate is slightly flattened by the longer weekend sessions, and it's a struggle to elevate it during these interval workouts. For these longer intervals it's perfectly acceptable to work in mid to upper Zone 3 and to almost view them as slightly shorter, sharper and faster tempo sessions. The most important thing is that your effort is consistent and you're working hard.

FRIDAY

In the previous blocks, you might have felt a bit frustrated by having to take a full day's rest, but you'll certainly appreciate it now. Put your feet up, put your compression tights on and enjoy having a workout-free day.

SATURDAY

As with the last block, we start with a long day out on the hills. Again, this is for a change of scenery and pace and to prove that you can last the time on your feet required for a marathon. It's then back into LSD runs that build up to three weekends in a row of two and a half hour efforts. Within these runs are specified time blocks of work in Zone 2. Try to work these into the middle of your run and to stay consistently in the middle of the zone. Obviously, running on a flat or gently undulating course will make this far easier. These efforts will get you used to running a strong focused pace at a precise intensity for prolonged periods. This is exactly what you'll need on marathon day, and practising eating and drinking without speeding up or slowing down is another skill you'll learn.

SUNDAY

Sticking predominately with the 90-minute cycle, follow the same protocol as in Level 3. Your legs will probably feel wretched when you first head out, so stick to a low gear and spin really easily. As your legs ease, build up the effort if you feel good, but keep things steady if they remain heavy.

CHAPTER 5

Level 5: The rest of your life

First, massive congratulations on your amazing achievement. Hopefully you really enjoyed your big day and achieved all the goals you'd set yourself. Despite the elation, and probably relief, of crossing the finish line, don't be surprised in the weeks following your marathon if you feel a bit down and demotivated. If you ask my wife, she'll tell you that I'm an absolute nightmare after big races. For so long your marathon has been a huge focal point in your life and now, it's over, losing that goal is bound to have an effect. This is perfectly normal and very common, but without taking it in hand it can make getting back into regular training very tough. People will commonly run a marathon and then not don their running shoes for six months, a year or even never again. This is such a shame, and a huge waste of an awful lot of hard work. In this final chapter we'll get you back into running post-marathon, and make suggestions as to what to focus on next.

Recovery Starts on the Finish Line

The temptation to collapse on crossing the line is understandable, but keeping moving for at least 10 minutes and then easing into some gentle stretching makes a massive difference to speed of recovery. As soon as you can stomach it, ideally within 15–20 minutes, drink a recovery drink containing carbohydrates and protein and then carry on sipping water. Put on some compression recovery tights and, once home, elevate your legs. Try to keep moving on a regular basis. A gentle 10–20 minute stroll in the evening is a good idea. Booking in for a massage can be helpful, but make it at least 72 hours post-race. Too soon and you'll be too sore to get maximum benefit from it.

PLAN YOUR RECOVERY

In the same way that you religiously planned your training, adopt a similar approach to your recovery. Full recovery from a marathon can take from four to six weeks, so see it as another training block. Without the discipline and the structured plan that's been such a big part of your life for so long, it's too easy to be haphazard in your approach and slip into sporadic and ineffective training. Not only will this prolong the recovery phase, but you'll be losing valuable fitness. Plan your recovery block before marathon day so it's set in stone and you have no excuses.

TAKE A CONSCIOUS BREAK FROM RUNNING

For a week, schedule in no running. Not only will this give you a physical break from the impact, but it'll also give you a mental break. After all, you've done quite a bit of running in the last few months. Cycling, swimming, upper body gym work, and yoga are all great options during this period. Keep intensity low but try to keep up a similar number of workouts as you did when marathon training to get you back into a regular training routine without losing momentum or motivation. Also, don't forget your friends and family. For months, running and training will have dominated every weekend, so take some time out to enjoy doing some normal non-running weekend activities.

FIRST RUNS BACK, NO PRESSURE

After a week, schedule in a run but make it really low key. Go to a favourite loop of road, trail or parkland that you know will take 15–30 minutes, ditch your watch and heart rate monitor, and just run. Focus on remembering what you enjoyed about running, and relish just getting back into it. End the session before you start to feel fatigued or before you stop enjoying it. Apply this length of run and lack of structure for your first three to five runs back. After two to three weeks you should have your running mojo back and be into a consistent training pattern. At this point you should start to reintroduce some structured tempo and interval sessions. Getting back into your strength routine will help to iron out any niggles or imbalances and prepare your body for harder training. Follow this four-week post-marathon plan that'll give you some time off but get you moving, running and back into training quickly and safely.

Four Weeks Post-Marathon

	Week 1	Week 2	Week 3	Week 4
Monday	Rest	Gym workout. Yoga/Pilates/ upper body	Gym workout. Yoga/Pilates/ upper body	Recovery session. Yoga/Pilates
Tuesday	Swim 30 mins	Run 1: 15–30 mins Zone 1	Run 1: 30–45 mins Zone 1–2 Followed by strength routine	Run 1: 30 mins tempo (10–**15**–5) Followed by strength routine
Wednesday	Massage	Swim 30 mins	Swim 30 mins	Swim 30 mins
Thursday	Cycle 30 mins Zone 1	Run 2: 15–30 mins Zone 1	Run 2: 25 mins tempo (10–**10**–5) Followed by strength routine	Run 2: Intervals 3 x 5 mins (3 mins reco) Followed by strength routine
Friday	Rest day	Rest day	Rest day	Rest day
Saturday	Cycle 30 mins Zone 1	Run 3: 15–30 mins Zone 1	Run 3: LSD 45 mins Zone 1–2	Run 3: LSD 60 mins Zone 1–2
Sunday	Family time	Family time	Cycle 45 mins	Cycle 60 mins

What Next?

As you're working through the recovery block, start thinking about where you want to take your fitness and what new goal you want to start working towards. You might think, having run a marathon, what can you possibly do next to match it, but with the level and all-round nature of the fitness you've built there is a whole range of possibilities open to you. The recovery block should have fired up your enthusiasm for structured training again, and you should be keen to set yourself a new goal. However it's not unusual post-marathon to be hesitant about committing yourself to another training plan. I genuinely believe it's a mistake to think that you'll manage to keep your fitness ticking over without a goal to aim for. Without a goal, you'll find yourself missing training sessions and falling into a routine of sporadic workouts. Not only will you find your fitness frustratingly slipping away but, without structure, balance and consistency, you're far more likely to pick up injuries. Set that goal, plan your training and keep moving forwards. Here are some suggestions for you.

GOING FASTER

It's very rare for a marathon first-timer to have a perfect run. You might feel you could have gone harder, that you didn't quite get your nutrition, hydration or pacing spot-on, or blew up in the closing miles. If you're a relative newcomer to running you might also feel that you simply haven't unlocked all your potential. If any of these are the case and you feel motivated to have another crack at 26.2 miles, use your now excellent endurance base to launch a campaign at another marathon. You'll be starting from a much stronger position, and if you focus on an autumn marathon, then training through the summer is far easier. After your recovery block, you'll be likely to have five to six months to prepare for your next attempt at the marathon. I'd suggest initially working back through Level 3, placing an emphasis on trying to run faster and stronger. This obviously applies to the tempo and interval workouts but also, on the Saturday LSD sessions, trying to stay in Zone 2 for the majority of the run will increase your overall speed. At the end of that block you should run a significantly faster half marathon, and this should set you up for repeating Level 4. If you find you have longer than eight weeks between finishing Level 3 and your marathon, simply work through the block and then repeat Week 26 until you are two weeks away from the race.

Another option, if you don't feel inclined to chase minutes over the marathon distance but want to keep running, is to try to run faster over shorter distances. Don't think that this is a soft option, as the training required for a fast 5 km, 10 km or half marathon is really tough. What you'll lose in distance you'll more than make up for in intensity. Working through Level 3 again, with an emphasis on increased speed, would be ideal preparation for a faster half marathon. However, if you're looking for a fast 5 km or 10 km, joining a local running club and taking part in some regular track sessions will really sharpen your top-end speed. Don't worry about not being fit or fast enough, as there will be groups to suit all levels. Quality speed workouts are almost impossible to do on your own, and having a coach and other runners around you on the track is guaranteed to spur you on to work much harder. Work through Level 3, but slot the track workout in either as an additional session on the Monday or as a replacement for your Tuesday or Thursday session. If you do this, use it to replace the intervals workout but keep the tempo run in your schedule. You also don't need to go beyond 90 minutes for your Saturday LSD run, but should work predominately in Zone 2.

GOING LONGER

Although often seen as the height of human endurance, a marathon is just a warm-up for ultra runners. An ultra is defined as any race longer than the 26.2 miles of a standard marathon. In fact, the original marathon run by Pheidippides from Athens to Sparta was an epic ultra at 250 km and is now relived annually in the Spartathlon race. Ultra running is as much about mindset as physical fitness. The mindset begins with the realization that 26.2 is just a number, not the limit of human endurance but actually a beginning. Ultras are becoming really popular as people look for challenges not just beyond 26.2 miles but also in some of the most inhospitable areas of the planet. Many people who've run a marathon aren't interested in trying to shave minutes off their PBs, realize that they're not physiologically suited to running faster, want to run off the beaten track, or just want to explore the limits of their endurance. You've got a great physical base already from your marathon training, so it's just a case of building mental toughness and learning pacing. The only limit then is your imagination. Having completed this plan and run a marathon, you're a far stronger runner than I was when I decided to become an ultra runner. Here's my story.

My first exposure to ultra running came in 1999 when, as a fresh-faced, newly qualified Personal Trainer, I came to London. I had retired from rugby after a number of injuries, and was doing a bit of running to keep my fitness ticking over. My slightly unhinged ex-Marine boss had signed up for the infamous MDS, or Marathon des Sables (a self-sufficient, 150 miles, six-day stage race over the Moroccan Sahara) and, as I followed his progress on-line, the embryonic sparks of an insane plan flashed in my mind. I had been thinking about doing the London Marathon the following year, but this looked much more fun. Blisters, sand, heavy pack, limited rations and 50 °C heat versus chugging round the streets of London in an anonymous hoard: the decision was made. I diligently drew up a training plan, and my metamorphosis into an ultra runner began. After nine months of training and a growing obsession with lightweight kit, my MDS was only a couple of months away.

With the MDS in April, my first true ultra was a 'training run' for it. It was a cold February morning, and getting off the train at Reading station I was mentally preparing myself for the 54-mile Reading–Shepperton Thames Meander Run. This was to be my longest training run, which I hoped, if successful, would serve me well for the 52-mile day four of the MDS. Meeting up with the rest of the runners, I found most were in training for the MDS and many were to become close friends. Not only does adversity bond you but you also get a lot of time to chat over the course of an ultra. I have many memories of that day: sucking knee-deep mud, losing the path in Windsor, a long mobile chat with my father in a dark field near Runnymead, and discovering that Staines isn't a nice place to run through at night. Oddly, the finish is a blur, but still etched clearly in my mind more than any other memory, is running through 26.2 miles feeling strong and just carrying on. That's when I became an ultra runner.

Without getting too mushy, the MDS was the most amazing thing I have ever done and a true turning-point in my life. There isn't space in this book for the full account of my race but the following extracts from my diary give a taste:

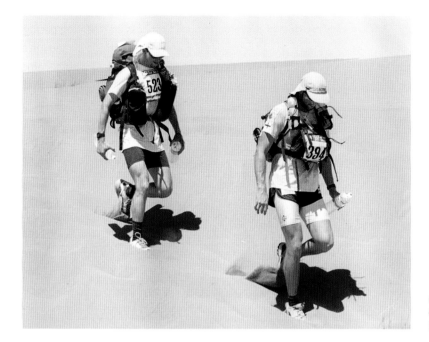

Slogging through the
dunes on the
Marathon des Sables

The size and steepness of the dunes made running up them impossible and a waste of valuable energy so John and I opted for walk up run down. At the bottom of each dune the air was still and roasting, it was like being in an oven. At the summit of each dune the breeze was welcome but the sight of dunes in every direction as far as the eye could see was truly daunting. After an hour in the dunes the three litres of water we picked up at the last checkpoint seemed woefully inadequate. Although we thought we were travelling painfully slowly we found we were working our way through the field and making steady, if slow, progress. At the top of one of the dunes we came across Kader. He was sat on his pack and looking bad. He was still lucid but obviously going downhill fast. We sat with him while we emptied our shoes of sand and ate a power bar. After trying to get him going he waved us off and, feeling more than a little guilty, we set off with him still sitting on his pack. Three hours into the dunes and I was starting to run low on water. Fortunately John, being a smaller build, wasn't getting through his so fast and in an act of huge generosity gave me an extra half litre. If I had been on my own and hadn't received these extra fluids I don't think I would have made it.

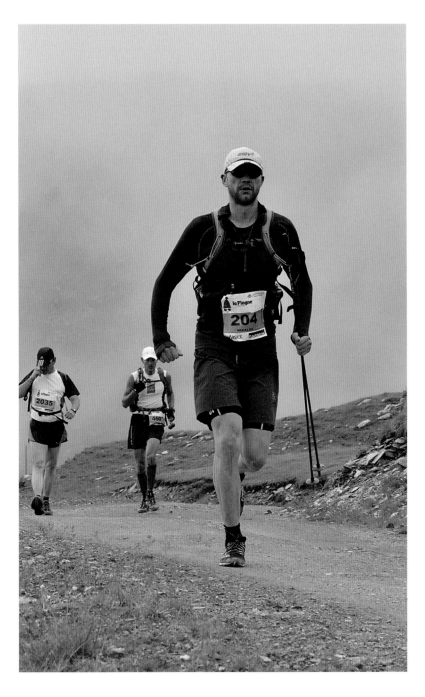

The author enjoying
a 60km trail race in
the French Alps

Marathon Training

After about 15 minutes my blood sugar crashed and I really started to struggle. I got tunnel vision and started to feel very dizzy; simply putting one foot in front of the other was a huge effort. Katie was in a similar state to me and Tessa was really suffering with bad feet. Fortunately Kath and John were still strong and dragged the rest of us through. Reaching the final checkpoint at 70 km we all made an effort to look as strong as possible so the medics wouldn't make us stop, we wanted to get this stage done as soon as we could.

The overwhelming emotion on crossing the line was pure relief. It was only on the coach back to Ouarzazate that the pride in what we achieved, and quite how badly we smelt, hit us. The Marathon des Sables has been the hardest thing I have ever done. The terrain and accumulative damage to your body makes it a huge challenge. You have to be physically fit but it really comes down to mental strength.

Since then, ultra running has taken me to the Himalayas, the Canadian Arctic and wonderful locations in Europe, and has allowed me to experience some of the wildest and most beautiful locations Britain has to offer. There is so much more to running than city centre marathons: look beyond the concrete, beyond 26.2, and you'll find a whole world of running adventures.

For training runs and low-key, low pressure events a great place to start is the Long Distance Walkers Association (LDWA). They organize a whole series of Challenge Walks covering distances from 20–100 miles, usually over mountainous, remote and rural locations. Entry fees are minimal, checkpoints often manned, and runners always welcome. *www.ldwa.org.uk*

✓ Montrail sponsor a 12-race ultra series taking in races from 30–61 miles all around the UK. The website is also an excellent resource for aspirant ultra runners. *www.runfurther.com*

✓ Another useful site, mainly for its comprehensive events list, is *www.ultrarunningworld.co.uk*

✓ For more exotic overseas events, EventRate is involved with some of the most prestigious ultra races in the world including the Yukon Arctic Ultra and the Jungle Marathon in the Amazon rainforest. *www.4ar.info*

✓ If you want to take on the Marathon des Sables, the UK agent for the race is The Best of Morocco. *www.saharamarathon.co.uk*. I've trained four people to successful completions of the Marathon des Sables, including two who had never run a marathon. None of them was an especially gifted runner, but by putting in consistent training they all achieved a truly amazing accomplishment. A training plan that follows the latter stages of Level 4 would be ideal initial preparation for an ultra. You would probably replace the tempo and intervals sessions with longer, steadier runs, building up to 90–120 minutes in Zones 1–2. You'd also need to make your Saturday LSD run longer and steadier. You should be looking to walk any uphills, jog flats and only really run when going downhill. Build up so that you're out on your feet for four to six hours, and try to train on hilly off-road terrain.

MULTISPORT

With the running, cycling and swimming fitness you've developed, another obvious direction to take your endurance base is into the world of multisport.

Triathlon, with its three disciplines, is probably one of the ultimate tests of all-round fitness. Training for it develops very balanced fitness and a great physique, and carries on with the low injury risk approach you've already been following. The great news is, having completed this programme, you're almost ready to attempt an Olympic-distance race. This consists of a 1500 m swim, a 40 km bike ride and a 10 km run. Also, if you ran a spring marathon, you're in the perfect position to race some triathlons over the summer.

Following a routine similar to Level 3, with a few minor alterations, will tweak your fitness ready for an Olympic-distance triathlon. Unless you come from a swimming background, your weakest discipline will probably be the swim. Remedy this by adding an extra swim on Monday to complement Wednesday's swim, and try to build up so that you're covering the 1,500 m in the session. Also consider having some additional technique coaching as, even more so than pure swimming fitness, a strong, economical and technically sound swimming stroke will make the biggest improvement to your swim leg. Both the tempo and intervals running workouts are applicable to a strong 10 km run at the end of a triathlon, but you only need to be running for up to

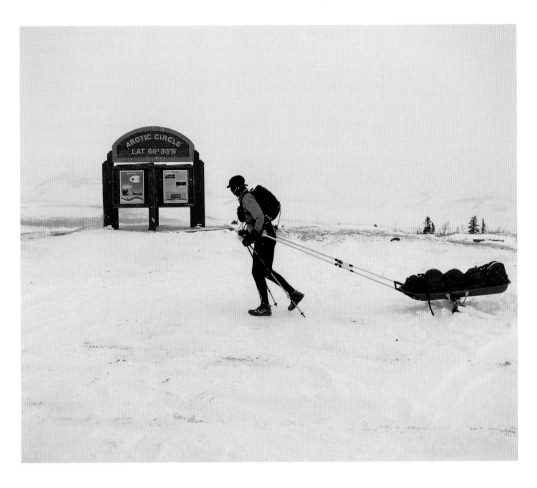

The author crossing the Arctic Circle during the 120-mile 6633 Ultra

90 minutes for your weekend LSD session. Continuing with your strength training will continue to safeguard you against injury and add functional strength for both running and cycling. You might also want to introduce some upper body movements such as bench presses, lat pull-downs and overhead presses to complement your swimming. You'll want to build your weekend cycle up to 120 minutes, and try to include two 20-minute Zone 2 consistent efforts into the ride. If you feel your cycling needs some additional work, replacing the intervals running workout with a spinning class is an ideal way to get a convienient high intensity bike session. Another good idea to prepare you for race day is to try to run straight off your weekend bike ride and/or the

spinning class. Known as a 'Brick Session', this gets you used to the jelly-legged sensation of running after a hard bike leg. You only need to run for 15–20 minutes, but aim to run at a tempo intensity. You'll find that your legs might feel weak and heavy for the first five to 10 minutes but quickly ease up as you settle into your running stride.

You can take part in a triathlon on any roadworthy bike, but to get the most out it a decent lightweight road bike is a good idea. If the triathlon bug really bites you might want to consider upgrading to an aerodynamic time trial-specific bike for race day and use your road bike for training. A cheaper option, to give yourself a bit of an aerodynamic edge, is to fit a pair of clip-on aerobars to your road bike. These simply bolt on to your handlebars and allow you to get into a low profile, wind-cheating tuck position.

After a few Olympic-distance races, you might start to toy with the idea of training for an Ironman triathlon. Don't forget you've already done the end discipline of an Ironman, but a marathon is a bit tougher on the back of a 3.8 km swim and a 180 km bike ride. If the idea appeals to you, a sensible approach after a summer of Olympic-distance races is to adopt a two-year plan. The next year would be spent training for and racing a few half Ironman distance races (1.9 km swim, 90 km bike ride, 20.1 km run) with a training load not a huge amount more than Olympic-distance preparation. Weekend LSD runs would creep up to 120 minutes, and you'd need to be completing regular three- to four-hour bike rides. Over the next winter you'd need to work predominately on building up your cycling fitness with regular rides of up to six hours. Long runs would increase to two and a half hours, and you'd be needing to spend significant time in the pool. The absolute minimum training commitment in the six to 12 months building up to an Ironman is 10 hours per week, but a more realstic volume is 15–20 hours.

Many people are put off the idea of a triathlon by the prospect of the swim leg, especially if it's an open water swim in a murky lake. Although pool-based events are fairly commonplace, an ideal way to dip your toe in the water of multisport is to do a duathlon. With a run–bike–run format, don't think that a duathlon is a soft touch. It's widely acknowledged among racers who do both triathlons and duathlons that the second run of the latter is tougher than the final run in the former. The duathlon season is split into two blocks, with races taking place in the autumn/early winter and then late winter/early spring. The

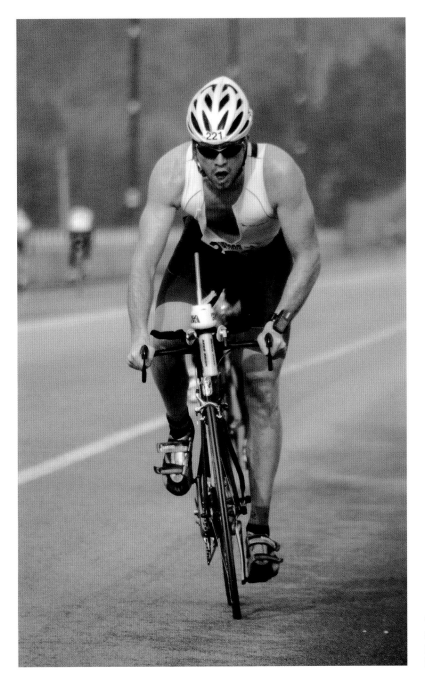

The author on the
bike leg of the
Powerman Malaysia
Duathlon

classic distances for a duathlon are 10 km–40 km–5 km. You'll also find half-distance sprint events and far longer. For those of you who like the rough stuff, there are plenty of off-road duathlons that combine mountain biking and trail running. The distances of these are usually shorter, and the biking, although usually muddy and hilly, doesn't tend to be overly technical. In fact, as most people have a serviceable mountain bike lurking in the garage, and as you don't have to worry about cars, an off-road event can be the perfect taster. Adopt a similar training approach as for an Olympic-distance triathlon but opt for an extra cycling session or a spinning class rather than Wednesday's swim.

For more information on triathlon and duathlon go to *www.britishtriathlon.org*

If you want more of a team challenge and don't mind the mud and wet, another option is the growing sport of Adventure Racing. Usually consisting of trail running, mountain biking, kayaking and some more unusual challanges, there are events to suit all levels. Go to *www.sleepmonsters.co.uk*

Index